A New Approach in the Treatment of Climacteric Disorders

New Developments in Biosciences 7

A New Approach in the Treatment of Climacteric Disorders

Editors
H. P. G. Schneider · A. R. Genazzani

Walter de Gruyter
Berlin · New York 1992

Deutsche Bibliothek — Cataloging-in-Publication Data

A new approach in the treatment of climacteric disorders / ed.: H. P. G. Schneider; A. R. Genazzani. — Berlin ; New York : de Gruyter, 1992
(New developments in biosciences ; 7)
ISBN 3-11-013471-3
NE: Genazzani, Andrea R. [Hrsg.]; GT

ISSN 0935-1906

Medical science is constantly developing. Research and clinical experience expand our knowledge, especially with regard to treatment and medication.

For dosages and applications mentioned in this work, the reader may rely on the authors, editors and publisher having taken great pains to ensure that these indications reflect the standard of knowledge at the time this work was completed.

Nevertheless, all users are requested to check the package leaflet of the medication, in order to determine for themselves whether the recommendations given for the dosages or the likely contraindications differ from those given in this book. This is especially true for medication which is seldom used or has recently been put on the market and for medication whose application has been restricted by the German Ministry of Health.

Typesetting and Printing: Arthur Collignon GmbH, Berlin. — Binding: Dieter Mikolai, Berlin. — Cover design: Rudolf Hübler, Berlin. — Printed in Germany.

Addresses

Editors

Prof. Dr. A. R. Genazzani
University Hospital of Modena
Department of Obstetrics
and Gynecology
Via del Pozzo 71
I-41100 Modena
Italy

Prof. Dr. H. P. G. Schneider
University of Münster
Department of Obstetrics
and Gynecology
Albert-Schweitzer-Str. 33
D-4400 Münster
Germany

List of first-mentioned contributors

Prof. Dr. C. Christiansen
Glostrup Hospital
University of Copenhagen
Department of Clinical Chemistry
DK-2600 Glostrup

Prof. Dr. A. R. Genazzani
University Hospital of Modena
Department of Obstetrics
and Gynecology
Via del Pozzo 71
I-41100 Modena

Prof. Dr. P. Koninckx
University Hospital
Gasthisberg-St. Rafael
Department of Obstetrics
and Gynecology
B-3000 Leuven

Prof. Dr. H. P. G. Schneider
University of Münster
Department of Obstetrics
and Gynecology
Albert-Schweitzer-Str. 33
D-4400 Münster

Prof. Dr. M. J. Tikkanen
Helsinki University Central Hospital
First Department of Medicine
Haartmaninkatu 4
SF-00290 Helsinki 29

Contents

Cyproterone acetate in hormone replacement therapy

C. Christiansen

Introduction

In 1900 the average life expectancy of women in the western part of the world was below 50 years; today it is 79 years. In the same period, the average age of menopause has been virtually unchanged. As we live longer, age related diseases become an increasing problem, as do diseases related to the menopause. Osteoporosis is a prime example. It is characterized by an age related and especially a menopause related universal, gradual, and relentless reduction in bone mass, which compromises the mechanical competence of the skeleton to such an extent that even minimal trauma may result in fracture. Figure 1 illustrates decrease in bone mass and increase in fracture incidence as a function of age in women, and demonstrates the rapid rise in fracture incidence which begins in the fourth decade in women. Figure 2 shows the distribution of fractures occurred after the menopause, and caused by minimal traumas, in a Danish population of 70-year old women. It appears that more than 40% of women at that age have had a fracture attributable to low bone mass.

Prevention of osteoporosis, rather than cure, is not only a more desirable, but probably a more realistic goal. The basis of preventive therapy lies in correction risk factors which the individual patient may demonstrate. Regarding postmenopausal osteoporosis there are a number of clinical factors which may represent risk factors, and the clinician must take these factors into account when estimating risk for each individual. After considering the possibilities of correcting these factors, the clinician and the patient have to decide on instituting estrogen substitution therapy. It is now established from long-term prospective studies that estradiol/progestogen therapy prevents postmenopausal bone loss from both peripheral and axial sites of the skeleton. Several epidemiological studies support that prevention of bone loss reduce fracture incidence. All the common estrogens, when used at appropriate dose, seem to be effective in preventing further bone loss. The optimal dose is for estradiol between 1 and 2 mg/day. Hormone treatment for prevention of osteoporosis must be maintained for a long period to ensure that bone mass will be sufficient

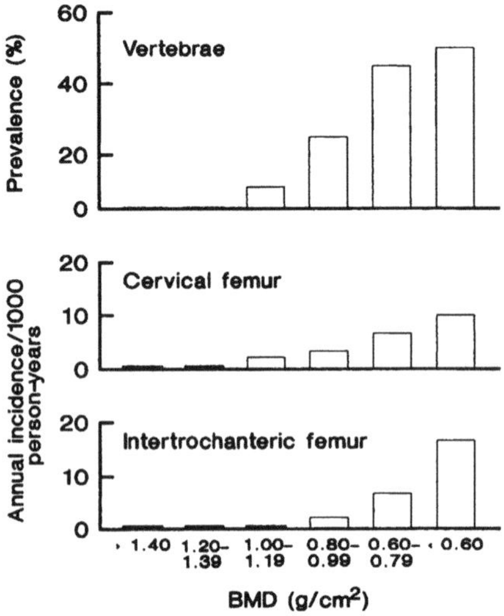

Fig. 1: Decrease in bone mass and increase in fracture incidence at different skeletal sites (Riggs, B. L., L. J. Melton III: Involutional osteoporosis. NEJM *314* (1986) 1676–1686, with permission).

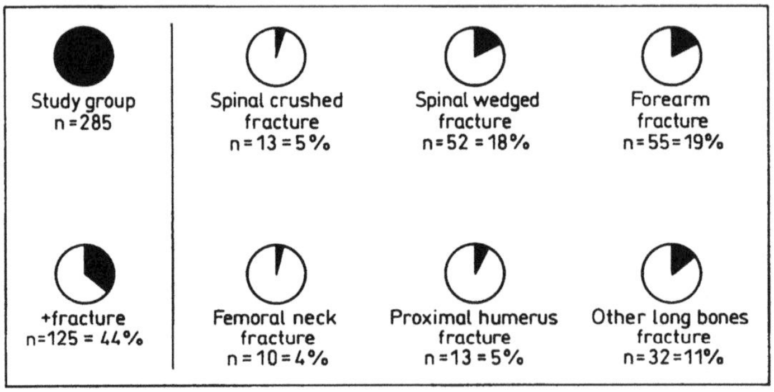

Fig. 2: Distribution of osteoporotic fractures in otherwise healthy women aged 70 years.

throughout life. Withdrawal of estrogen therapy results in a rate of bone loss parallel to that just after menopause, i. e. the beneficial effect is life-long, and not lost in a few years because of an acceleration of bone loss (Fig. 3).

Treatment for longer periods with unopposed estrogen increases the risk of endometrial hyperplasia, whereas addition of a progestogen seems to eliminate this. Combined estrogen/progestogen therapy has, therefore, become an essen-

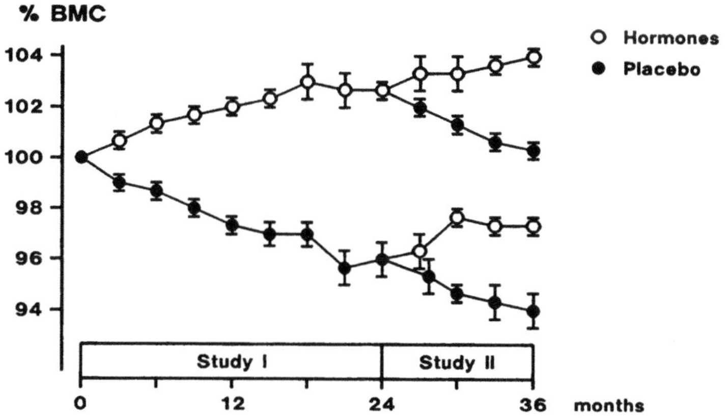

Fig. 3: Bone mass in postmenopausal women during treatment with hormone replacement therapy (o) and placebo (•), and after withdrawal. The rate of bone loss after withdrawal is similar to that seen after a normal menopause (Christiansen, C., M. S. Christensen, I. Transbøl: Bone mass in postmenopausal women after withdrawal of oestrogen/gestagen replacement therapy. Lancet *I* (1981) 459–461, with permission).

tial feature of postmenopausal hormone substitution therapy. Progestogens derived from 19-nor-testosterone have androgenic properties and may adversely affect the lipid metabolism, whereas this may not be the case for the hydroxy-progesterone derivatives.

In search of a proper and safe progestogen for postmenopausal hormone replacement therapy, we studied the effects of a cyclic combination of estradiol valerate (EV), and the anti-androgenic progestogen cyproterone acetate (CPA) on bone mass [4], serum lipids and lipoproteins [3], bleeding pattern [3], blood pressure [1], and climacteric symptoms [2] in a double-blind placebo-controlled trial.

Patients and methods

65 healthy early postmenopausal women were allocated to treatment with either EV (2 mg) (day 1–21) + CPA (1 mg) (day 12–21) or placebo, and were examined at 3-month intervals for 2 years.

Bone mineral content was measured in the forearms by single photon absorptiometry, in the lumbar spine and in the total skeleton by dual photon absorptiometry.

Serum total cholesterol, HDL-cholesterol, and *triglycerides* were measured by standard procedures in our laboratory, and *LDL-cholesterol* was estimated according to Friedewald et al. Biochemical estimates of bone turnover, i. e. *serum alkaline phosphatase, phosphate, fasting urinary calcium* and *hydroxyproline* were measured by standard procedures.

Bleeding records were obtained from the participants who filled in a calendar for daily registration of tablet intake and vaginal bleeding. *Climacteric symptoms* were obtained using the menopausal index of Kupperman.

Results

Forearm bone mass: In the group treated with EV/CPA the mean values of the measurements at all examinations remained unchanged from the initial values. Linear regression analysis was performed on the values of each individual versus time, and the mean slope was not significantly different from zero. In the group treated with placebo the mean forearm bone mass values gradually declined with time, reaching a value of about 95% at two years, which was highly significantly different from the mean value of the hormone group. Linear regression analysis showed a rate of bone loss from this area of approximately 2.5% per year (5% over 2 years) (Fig. 4).

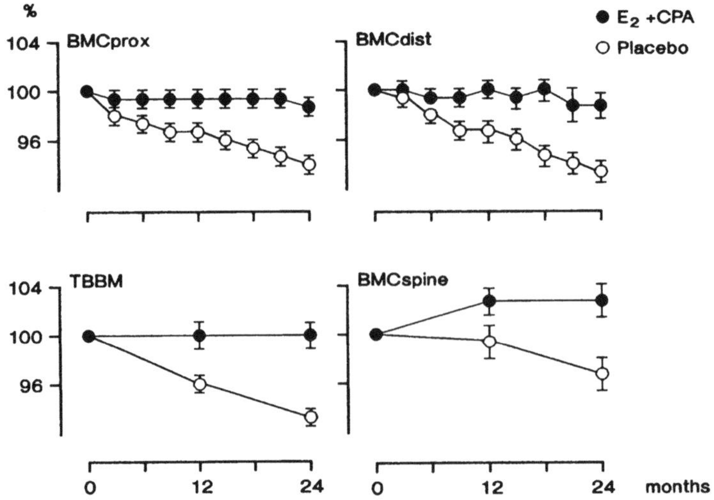

Fig. 4: Bone mass in the forearms (BMC arm) spine (BMD spine) and total skeleton (TBBM) during 24 months treatment with cyclical EV/CPA (•) or placebo (o). (From Riis et al. [4] with permission)

Total body bone mineral (TBBM): The mean values of the TBBM measurements in the group treated with EV/CPA remained unchanged throughout the trial. In the placebo group there was an almost linear decrease in TBBM with time; the mean values at 12 and 24 months were both significantly different from the hormone group. Rate of bone loss, was approximately 3.5% per year (7% per 2 years) (Fig. 4).

Spinal bone mass: Owing to a much larger variance of this method (5%), comparison of the mean values in the two groups with their respective initial values is meaningless. Comparison of the EV/CPA group with the placebo group, however, showed a gradually increasing difference between the two groups during the study, thus reaching a highly significant difference of about 6% at 2 years (Fig. 4).

Biochemical estimates of bone formation (serum alkaline phosphatase, plasma BGP, and 95-UE): In the hormone group serum alkaline phosphatase decreased after institution of treatment, reaching about 15% at 6 months and falling to a level 75% of the initial value during the remaining part of the study. The placebo group showed a minor increase of 10% in serum alkaline phosphatase over the two years. The difference between the two groups at two years was highly significant. Plasma BGP had decreased rapidly to about 50% of the initial values at 3 months of hormone treatment and remained virtually at that level throughout the trial. In the placebo group the mean values of BGP at any of the examination times were not significantly different from the initial values. The differences between the two treatment groups at two years was highly significant. 95-UE showed a highly significant decrease to a premenopausal level in the hormone group, whereas it remained virtually unchanged in the placebo group throughout the study.

Biochemical estimates of bone resorption (serum phosphate, fasting urinary calcium/creatinine, and hydroxyproline/creatinine): In the hormone group all the bone resorption parameters decreased significantly during the two years of treatment. The changes generally reached their maximum within the first 6 months. In the placebo group the biochemical estimates of bone resorption remained virtually unchanged at a high level during the two years.

Effects on serum concentration of lipoproteins: Total serum cholesterol and LDL-cholesterol in the hormone group were reduced at all examinations, whereas virtually no changes were observed in the placebo group. Although serum triglycerides tended to increase during hormone treatment, the rise was not significantly different from that in the placebo group. Both groups showed almost constant HDL-cholesterol levels during the first 6 months and slight increases during the last 6 months (Fig. 5). The cumulative response on serum lipids and lipoproteins in the hormone group showed significantly reduced levels of total cholesterol and LDL-cholesterol, whereas the minor increases

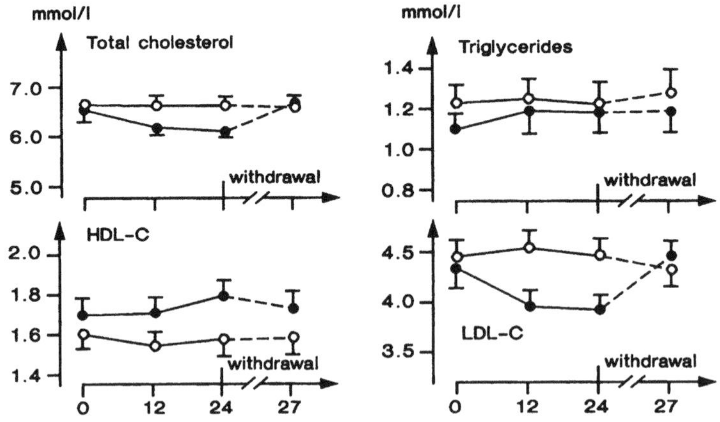

Fig. 5: Serum lipids and lipoproteins during 24 months treatment with cyclical EV/CPA (•) or placebo (o). (From Jensen et al. [3] with permission)

observed in serum triglycerides and HDL-cholesterol were not statistically significant. The cumulative response with placebo was not significantly different from the initial values in either of the variables.

Effects on safety parameters: No significant changes were seen in hemoglobin, serum creatinine, on serum aspartate aminotransferase (ASAT), in either of the two treatment groups during the trial.

Blood pressure and body weight: The diastolic blood pressure tended to increase with time in the placebo group when compared with the hormone group, but the difference was significant only at 18 and 21 months. Likewise, the cumulated response on blood pressure showed a tendency toward increased diastolic blood pressure in the placebo group when compared with the hormone group. The difference did not, however, become significant. Correlations between the mean values of diastolic and systolic blood pressure and time were insignificant in the hormone group. In the placebo group there was a positive and significant correlation between both diastolic and systolic blood pressure and time.

The mean body weight remained unchanged throughout the trial in the hormone group, whereas an average weight increase was seen in the placebo group.

Kupperman index: The number of subjective menopausal symptoms (Kupperman index) decreased significantly in the hormone group to a level not different from that of premenopausal women. In the placebo group the Kupperman index remained unchanged.

Vaginal bleeding: In the hormone group 27 women (73%) ecperienced minor regular bleeding during each tablet pause, whereas 8 women only occasionally had vaginal bleeding during the tablet pause. One participant did not experience any bleeding at all, and one woman, who had considerable and irregular bleeding, had a biopsy taken; cytology showed no abnormality. Five women (13%) in the placebo group experienced one minor vaginal bleeding within the first 2 months of the study. None of the participants were withdrawn from or left the trial, because of hormone induced metrorrhagia. The bleeding pattern gives an estimate of the condition of the endometrium but may not replace endometrial biopsy, which was not included in the present study.

Side-effects: Two participants left the study (within three months) for medical reasons: one because of varicose veins developed in the legs and one because of a weight increase (both were in the hormone group). The relation to the treatment is not clear. Four participants left the study because of unacceptable subjective menopausal symptoms (all were in the placebo group). None of the participants developed carcinoma of the breast or the endometrium. No untoward cardiovascular reactions were observed.

Conclusions

The results of the present study may be summarized as follows:

- Treatment with EV/CPA prevents postmenopausal bone loss from all parts of the skeleton.
  Biochemical estimates showed that bone formation and resorption are "normalized" to a premenopausal level during treatment with hormone.
- Body weight and blood pressure were unchanged during treatment, in contrast to the placebo group where a significant increase was found in both parameters.
- Subjective menopausal symptoms (the Kupperman index) decrease to a level not significantly different from that in premenopausal women.
- Most of the women experienced regular menstrual bleeding.
- No serious side-effects were observed.

References

[1] Hassager, C., B. J. Riis, V. Strøm, et al.: The long-term effect of oral and percutaneous estradiol on plasma renin substrate and blood pressure. Circulation *76* (1987) 753–758.

[2] Jensen, P. B., J. Jensen, B. J. Riis, et al.: Climacteric symptoms after oral and percutaneous hormone replacement therapy. Maturitas *9* (1987) 207–215.

[3] Jensen, J., B. J. Riis, V. Strøm, et al.: Long-term and withdrawal effects of two different oestrogen-progestogen combinations on lipid and lipoprotein profiles in postmenopausal women. Maturitas *11* (1989) 117–128.

[4] Riis, B. J., Jensen, J., C. Christiansen: Cyproterone acetate, an alternative gestagen in postmenopausal estrogen/gestagen therapy. Clin. Endocrinol. *26* (1987) 327–334.

Combination of estradiol-valerate and cyproterone acetate – a modern regimen for hormone replacement therapy

M. J. Tikkanen

Introduction

There is increasing evidence mainly from observational studies indicating that postmenopausal estrogen replacement therapy is effective in preventing coronary heart disease (CHD). Most of the evidence is based on studies carried out using estrogen alone. Modern treatment regimens contain, in addition, cyclic progestin creating a need to develop combined hormone preparations which preserve the effect of estrogen on CHD risk. Accordingly, there is a search going on for progestin components which will not counteract the favorable effects of estrogen on serum lipid and lipoprotein risk factors and which will be well tolerated by women. This paper provides a short introduction to this field, and the results of a pilot study employing estradiol valerate in cyclic combination with cyproterone acetate will be reported.

Background

Hormone replacement therapy and serum lipid risk factors for coronary heart disease

It is well established that estrogen administered alone has beneficial effects on the serum lipid and lipoprotein profile. This is particularly evident in women with initially high cholesterol levels such as the postmenopausal Finnish women reported in 1978 [16] who represented a population with an average serum cholesterol level of about 8.5 mmol/l. In that study low density lipoprotein (LDL) cholesterol was reduced by 18% and high density lipoprotein (HDL) cholesterol increased by approximately 30% by estradiol valerate 2 mg/d with no significant change in serum triglyceride levels. However, a combination of levonorgestrel with the estradiol regimen in a later study resulted in marked reductions in HDL-cholesterol, which were due to the reduction in the HDL2 subfraction [15]. As progestin addition is essential for women who have not undergone hysterectomy, studies were initiated to characterize progestin components which would counteract the effects of estrogens on the lipoprotein profiles as little as possible. To evaluate the androgenicity of progestins, we employed the measurement of hepatic lipase activity in postheparin plasma. In a series of studies we observed that this enzyme activity was stimulated by progestins with inherent androgenic properties, but not by progestins which were relatively non-androgenic. Moreover, increases in hepatic lipase activity were always associated with decreases in HDL2-cholesterol levels providing a means of predicting the effects of any given progestin on HDL-cholesterol. Preliminary studies were carried out with progestins such as medroxyprogesterone acetate [14], desogestrel [9], and cyproterone acetate [13], indicating that these steroids were less androgenic than levonorgestrel and that only minor effects, if any, on hepatic lipase and on HDL-cholesterol levels occurred with the dosages used.

These initial results suggested that combinations with estrogen using such progestins might preserve the estrogen-induced effects on serum lipid and lipoprotein risk factors for CHD and might, at least in theory, provide protection against CHD.

Hormone replacement therapy and coronary heart disease

Epidemiologic evidence is accumulating which strongly suggests that estrogen use in postmenopausal women protects against cardiovascular disease (Tab. 1) [1]. Various types of prospective cohort studies, case-control or population-controlled studies, and more recently studies also employing coronary angiography have been reported. The most recent major epidemiologic study [11] indicated that the risk of coronary heart disease was reduced to one half in

Table 1: Estrogen use in women and risk of cardiovascular disease (Summary of 24 published reports up to 1991)

	Risk estimate*		
Design of study	≤ 0.80	0.81 – 1.05	> 1.05
Angiographic (case-control or cross-sectional)	3		
Cohort	7		1
Case-control	4	2	3
Clinical trial	1		
Population-controlled	3		

* Statistically significant reductions in CHD risk by approx. 50% were demonstrated in 11 out of 24 published reports (adapted from [1]).

women currently taking estrogen as compared to estrogen non-users. Only one prospective study has suggested an increase in coronary heart disease [17]. This result was obtained in the Framingham cohort, and has been subjected to reanalysis recently [3]. The new analysis was carried out in order to make the results comparable to other studies (for example, excluding angina pectoris as an endpoint). It revealed that there was in fact protection against fatal CHD in women who were in their fifties and no association in women in their sixties, if they were taking estrogen. The majority of the evidence from the epidemiologic studies indicates that a risk reduction of about 50% can be demonstrated in women receiving estrogen replacement therapy. In a recent angiographic study [12] it was demonstrated that women who had severe coronary artery disease (stenosis of more than 70% in the coronary vessels or above 50% in the left main stem) benefited most from estrogen treatment. During a 10-year follow-up period, the survival of estrogen non-users became with time progressively less in comparison to estrogen users.

The mechanisms underlying the protective actions of estrogen against coronary heart disease have not been adequately explained. Some published reports have made indirect estimates about the role of reducing LDL-cholesterol and increasing HDL-cholesterol in CHD risk reduction [4, 2]. The reports suggested that modification of these lipoprotein risk factors could explain 25 to 50% of the beneficial effects of estrogen. This implies that 50 to 75% of the protective efficacy of estrogen has other explanations. These could include direct hemodynamic effects, and effects on coagulation and fibrinolytic parameters. Also many other mechanisms are possible.

Materials and methods

Design of the study

This pilot study was designed to compare the effects of estradiol valerate combined with cyproterone acetate with those of estradiol valerate alone. 13 postmenopausal women volunteered for the study. They were aged 56.5 ± 6.5 years (mean $\pm$ SD). No dietary instructions were given.

The baseline lipid and lipoprotein levels were measured twice and the averages of these determinations were used as baseline values. For at least three consecutive cycles, the participants received estradiol valerate 2 mg daily during cycle days 1–21 followed by a 7-day treatment pause. Six of the women received this estradiol regimen for 6 months. After this, all women received, in addition to estradiol valerate, cyproterone acetate (1 mg/d) during days 12–21 during one or more cycles. Five of the women volunteered to continue this combined regimen for 12 months. Serum lipid and lipoprotein determinations were carried out at baseline, after one and three cycles of estradiol alone, after the first cycle of the combined regimen with estradiol valerate and cyproterone acetate, as well as in five women after 3, 6 and 12 months using the combined regimen. The blood samples were drawn on day 21 ($\pm$ 1 day).

Methods

Very low density lipoprotein (VLDL) and LDL were isolated by sequential ultracentrifugation [5] in a Sorvall-OTD-2 ultracentrifuge at solvent densities of 1.006 and 1.063 g/ml for 18 and 24 h, respectively. The cholesterol concentrations were determined according to the method of Röschlau et al. [10] using a commercial kit (Boehringer Mannheim, F. R. G.). The triglyceride concentrations were analyzed in a Technicon Autoanalyzer II (Technicon Instruments, Tarrytown, NY, U. S. A.) [8].

Post-heparin blood was drawn 15 minutes after an intravenous injection of 100 IU (1 mg) of sodium heparin (Medica, Helsinki, Finland) per kg body weight. Determinations of hepatic lipase and lipoprotein lipase (LPL) activity in post-heparin plasma were carried out using a specific immunochemical method [6].

Results

The main results are presented in Table 2 and Figure 1. Treatment with estradiol valerate 2 mg/d alone resulted in average reductions in serum cholesterol and LDL-cholesterol by 8% and 13%, respectively. There was little change in serum triglyceride and HDL-cholesterol levels. When cyproterone acetate was added to the regimen following the cycles of estrogen alone, slightly but not

Table 2: Serum lipid and lipoprotein levels in 13 postmenopausal women during hormone replacement therapy with estradiol valerate (2 mg/d) alone and in combination with cyproterone acetate 1 mg/d)*

mmol/l	Baseline	E_2V (3 cycles)	E_2V + CPA (1 cycle)
Cholesterol	6.19 $\pm$ 0.68	5.71 $\pm$ 0.94**	5.51 $\pm$ 0.67**
LDL-cholesterol	4.21 $\pm$ 0.73	3.65 $\pm$ 0.97**	3.48 $\pm$ 0.76**
Triglyceride	1.44 $\pm$ 0.53	1.46 $\pm$ 0.73	1.33 $\pm$ 0.53
HDL-cholesterol	1.74 $\pm$ 0.33	1.79 $\pm$ 0.40	1.77 $\pm$ 0.38

* Serum lipid and lipoprotein determinations were carried out on day 21 of the cycle.

** $p < 0.001$ (paired t-test vs. baseline)

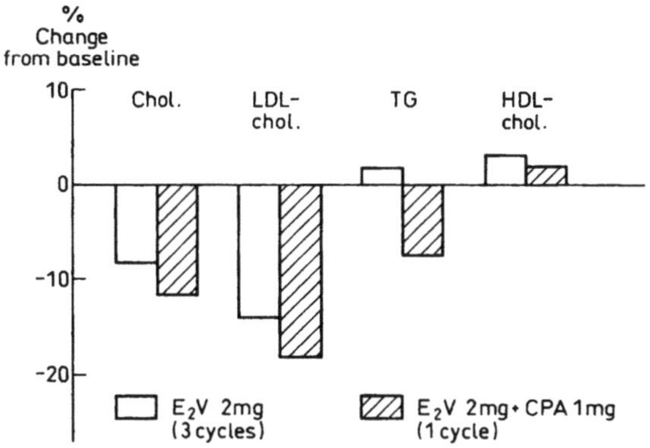

Fig. 1: Changes from baseline in serum lipoprotein lipids during estradiol valerate (2 mg/d) and after adding cyclic cyproterone acetate (1 mg/d).

significantly greater reductions were observed in cholesterol, LDL-cholesterol and also triglyceride levels.

Postheparin plasma lipase activities were assayed in 10 out of the 13 women participating in the study. The mean values for hepatic lipase during baseline, the third estradiol valerate cycle and during the combined regimen were 14.0 ± 4.5, 10.3 ± 3.4 and 10.2 ± 4.5 FFA $\mu mol \cdot h^{-1} \cdot ml^{-1}$, respectively. None of the differences between the means were statistically significant, nor was there any statistically significant variation in lipoprotein lipase activity (data not shown). The triglyceride/cholesterol ratios in LDL were also calculated in order to demonstrate whether estrogen treatment caused enrichment of triglyceride in LDL. However, there was only non-significant variation ranging from 0.10 ± 0.02 during baseline, 0.12 ± 0.04 during estradiol valerate and 0.13 ± 0.03 during combined treatment.

Five of the women volunteered to continue the estrogen-progestin combination for 12 months. Comparison of the serum lipid and lipoprotein levels between the first cycle with this regimen and the values obtained after one year indicated essentially no change apart from a slight increasing trend in HDL-cholesterol (1.65 mmol/l) after the first cycle to 1.72 mmol/l after one year.

Discussion

The present study was carried out in order to see whether addition of cyproterone acetate, a non-androgenic progestin, would counteract the effects of estradiol valerate on serum lipids and lipoproteins. The results indicate that the reductions in total and LDL-cholesterol were not impaired by addition of this progestin. Nor was HDL-cholesterol reduced during the combined regimen. However, one must exert some caution in interpreting the results. The study was designed to be a pilot study without a placebo group and the number of participants was small which could have influenced the results. However, similar changes from baseline for serum lipids have been reported previously using the same estrogen-progestin combination [7].

In a previous study in menstruating women [13] we demonstrated that postheparin plasma hepatic lipase activity was not increased by cyproterone acetate 5 mg/d. This suggested to us that using an even smaller dose (1 mg/d) of cyproterone acetate combined with estrogen would probably not reduce HDL-cholesterol levels. As expected, there was no change in postheparin plasma hepatic lipase activity and no reduction in HDL-cholesterol in the present study. This indicates that when added to estradiol valerate 2 mg daily, cyproterone acetate 1 mg daily does not produce an "androgenic" effect resulting in HDL-cholesterol reduction.

If one assumes that a significant part of the protection against CHD by estrogen therapy is mediated by changes in serum lipid risk factors, one may assume that this effect is not reduced by adding cyclic cyproterone acetate 1 mg/d. With respect to the serum lipoprotein profile, this combination appears to be favorable. However, there are many other factors contributing to the risk of atherosclerotic disease which have not been studied adequately. For example, the effects of this combination on coagulation and fibrinolytic factors, direct effects on the vessel walls, effects of the prostacyclin-thromboxane system, glucose tolerance and blood pressure have not been studied in detail. Further studies are therefore necessary to determine the effect of new estrogen-progestin combinations, such as the present combination of estradiol valerate and cyproterone acetate, on the overall risk of coronary heart disease in postmenopausal women.

References

[1] Barrett-Connor, E., T. L. Bush: Estrogen and coronary heart disease in women. JAMA *265* (1991) 1861–1867.

[2] Bush, T., E. Barrett-Connor, L. D. Cowan et al.: Cardiovascular mortality and non-contraceptive estrogen use in women: results from the Lipid Research Clinic's Program Follow-Up Study. Circulation *75* (1987) 1002–1009.

[3] Eaker, E. D., W. P. Castelli: Differential risk for coronary heart disease among women in the Framingham Study. In: E. Eaker, B. Packard, N. Wenger et al.: (eds.): Coronary heart disease in women, pp. 122–130. Haymarket Doyma, New York, NY 1987.

[4] Gruchow, H. W., A. J. Anderson, J. J. Barboriak et al.: Postmenopausal use of estrogen and occlusion of coronary arteries. Am. Heart J. *115* (1988) 954–963.

[5] Havel, R. J., H. A. Eder, J. H. Bragdon: The distribution and chemical composition of ultracentrifugally separated lipoproteins in human serum. J. Clin. Invest. 34 (1955) 1345–1353.

[6] Huttunen, J. K., C. Ehnholm, P. K. J. Kinnunen et al.: An immunochemical assay method for the selective measurement of two triacylglycerol lipases in human postheparin plasma. Clin. Chim. Acta *63* (1975) 335–347.

[7] Jensen, J. B., J. Riis, V. Strom et al.: Long-term and withdrawal effects of two different oestrogen-progestogen combinations on lipid and lipoprotein profiles in post-menopausal women. Maturitas *11* (1989) 117–128.

[8] Kessler, G., H. Lederer: Fluorimetric determination of triglycerides. In: L. T. Skeggs (ed.): Automation in analytical chemistry, p. 345. Mediad, New York 1965.

[9] Kuusi, T., E. A. Nikkilä, M. J. Tikkanen et al.: Effects of two progestins with different androgenic properties on hepatic endothelial lipase and high density lipoprotein$_2$. Atherosclerosis *54* (1985) 251–262.

[10] Röschlau, P., E. Bernt, W. Gruber: Enzymatische Bestimmung des gesamten Cholesterins im Serum. J. Clin. Chem. Clin. Biochem. *12* (1974) 403–408.

[11] Stampfer, M. J., G. A. Colditz, W. C. Willett et al.: Postmenopausal estrogen therapy and cardiovascular disease. Ten-year follow-up from the Nurses' Health Study. N. Eng. J. Med. *325* (1991) 756–762.

[12] Sullivan, J. M., R. V. Zwaag, G. F. Lemp et al.: Postmenopausal estrogen use and coronary atherosclerosis. Ann. Int. Med. *108* (1988) 358–363.

[13] Tikkanen, M. J., T. Kuusi, E. A. Nikkilä et al.: Postheparin plasma hepatic lipase activity as predictor of high density lipoprotein response to progestin therapy: studies with cyproterone acetate. Maturitas *9* (1987) 81–86.

[14] Tikkanen, M. J., E. A. Nikkilä, T. Kuusi et al.: Different effects of two progestins on plasma high density lipoprotein (HDL_2) and postheparin plasma hepatic lipase activity. Atherosclerosis *40* (1981) 365–369.

[15] Tikkanen, M. J., E. A. Nikkilä, T. Kuusi et al.: High density lipoprotein-2 and hepatic lipase: Reciprocal changes produced by estrogen and norgestrel. J. Clin. Endocrinol. Metab. *54* (1982) 1113–1117.

[16] Tikkanen, M. J., E. A. Nikkilä, E. Vartiainen: Natural oestrogen as an effective treatment for type-II hyperlipoproteinaemia in postmenopausal women. Lancet *II* (1978) 490–491.

[17] Wilson, P. W. F., R. J. Garrison, W. P. Castelli: Postmenopausal estrogen use and heart disease. N. Eng. J. Med. *315* (1986) 135.

Clinical experiences with a non-androgenic progestogen in an estradiol-valerate-containing regimen for hormone replacement therapy

H. P. G. Schneider, K. Schmidt-Gollwitzer

Introduction

The effective relief of distressing climacteric and postmenopausal symptoms is essentially based upon the prescription of one or another form of estrogen treatment. Progestogen monotherapy or the addition of progestogens to the estrogen regimen had been a domain of the treatment of cycle disturbances.

When estradiol valerate was sequentially combined with norgestrel, almost 15 years ago, it was originally designed to control cycle irregularities in the perimenopausal period and to provide an effective relief of typical climacteric complaints. Treatment at that time was restricted to a short-term intervention with a continuing check of the necessity for treatment.

The evidence of a preventive potency of estrogen replacement therapy with respect to postmenopausal osteoporosis, had changed the strategy for hormone replacement therapy (HRT) towards a long-term substitution. This substitution should now continue beyond the relief of symptoms and bleeding problems for 5 years and more.

The following presentation compares the progestagens norgestrel and cyproterone acetate as part of a treatment regimen with estradiol valerate for hormone replacement therapy. First, the rationale for the treatment regimen is discussed. Then, some results of the clinical investigation will be presented, focussing on symptom relief, bleeding pattern and some laboratory findings.

The treatment regimen

Estradiol valerate is the 17β-estradiol in form of a prodrug. The fatty acid is immediately split off after intestinal resorption leaving us with the "real" human estrogen. The Schering Company has had many years of experience with this estrogen. Its efficacy in HRT has already been documented with the investigations and the success of many preparations, e. g. Progynova, Cyclo-Progynova and others. The pharmacokinetics and all active metabolites are known. Furthermore, the influence of the human estradiol on liver metabolism is undoubtedly more physiological than that of conjugated, equine estrogens.

We feel therefore, that with the introduction of a preparation containing natural estrogens we have more than only an alternative to the widespread use of conjugated estrogens.

The cyclical addition of progestogens to an estrogen substitution in non-hysterectomized women to oppose estrogen influence on the endometrium is being practiced in many countries, and combination products have been available in Europe for several years.

There is currently no recommendation in the US labelling of estrogen products that adjuvant therapy with progestogens should be used, and no estrogen/progestogen combination products in the form of a "calendar pack" have been approved for US marketing. However, the US FDA's fertility and maternal health drugs advisory committee agreed that, despite the absence of long-term data on the use of any progestogen with estrogen therapy, enough data exist to recommend the addition of a progestogen on an individualised basis in the labelling of all estrogen products to reduce the risk of endmetrial cancer.

Fixed combinations have important advantages to simplify the treatment and to assure proper compliance to the regimen. Therefore, they may even be safer than individually composed treatment regimens.

There is the benefit of preventing endometrial hyperplasia and subsequently a reduced risk of endometrial carcinoma, but on the other hand, we also risk the reverse of the beneficial effect of estrogens on lipid metabolism, thereby increasing the risk of cardiovascular diseases.

There are two different classes of progestogens, the 19-Nor-testosterone derivates and the 17-OH-progesterone derivates:

19-nor-testosterone derivates appear to have a negative influence on lipid metabolism because of their partial androgenic activity. The estrogen-induced beneficial increase in the HDL/LDL-cholesterol ratio can be reversed in a dose-dependent manner. Consequently there is the risk of losing the possible prophylactic potency of HRT for cardiovascular diseases.

17-OH-progesterone derivatives have a lower androgenic activity in relation to their progestogenic potency than 19-nor-testosterone derivates. However, in higher dosages they are also able to counteract the estrogen influence on the lipoprotein pattern through their antiestrogenic potency. This, for example, would explain the HDL-lowering effect of medroxyprogesteroneacetate (MPA) in a daily dose of 10 mg, as was demonstrated by Ottosson, Johansson and von Schoultz [2].

The most commonly used progestins have androgenic properties with the potential of a negative influence on lipid metabolism. In particular, there is a lack of fixed combinations for HRT with hydroxyprogesterone derivates.

This has led to the introduction of cyproterone acetate (CPA) for the estradiol valerate substitution therapy. CPA derives from 17-OH-progesterone, is highly progestagenic and has no androgenic properties. From a certain dosage onwards it even exerts antiandrogenic activities.

Studies on its metabolic influences by Tikkanen et al. proved that CPA has no direct influence on the hepatic lipase activity in contrast to 19-nor-testosterone derivatives [4]. Hence, should the estrogen substitution therapy improve the lipoprotein pattern, we would expect the addition of CPA not to counteract this beneficial effect.

Cyclo-Progynova consists of 11 tablets with 2 mg estradiol valerate and 10 tablets with 2 mg estradiol valerate plus 0.5 mg norgestrel. This preparation was introduced to the German market about 15 years ago.

Climen is a preparation with 21 days of 2 mg estradiol valerate and a 10-day addition of 1 mg cyproterone per day. The regimen is followed by a 7-day interval of no tablet intake (Fig. 1). The design of Clivian is adopted from Cyclo-Progynova. A reccurence of complaints within the 7 days of no tablet intake was not reported in any of our clinical studies.

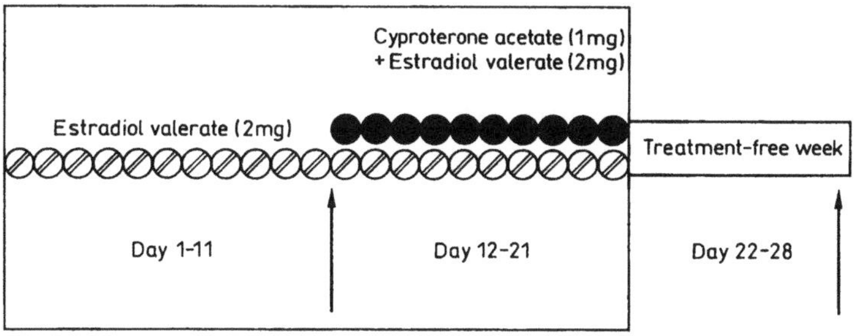

Fig. 1: Climen-intake regimen

Thus both preparations follow an identical regimen. The only difference constitutes in the progestational compound. Cyclo-Progynova contains norgestrel, a 17-nortestosterone derivative, whereas Climen combines estradiol valerate with cyproterone acetate, a 17-OH-progesterone derivative for 10 days.

Patients and methods

A randomized, double-blind, multi-centre study has been performed to compare the clinical efficacy of both preparations. On completion of the study, 594 patients were included in the evaluation, 293 of them had received Climen and 301 Cyclo-Progynova. The duration of the trial had been set for 12 treatment cycles.

The objective of the trial was to compare the clinical efficacy and bleeding pattern of the two different preparations. Laboratory determinations were performed by Prof. Hirvonen, University of Helsinki and recently published [1]. Later on, these results will shortly be summarized.

Table 1 gives the age distribution of the study population, the percentage of pre- and postmenopausal women and the duration of menopausal complaints. According to the inclusion criteria only patients with typical climacteric complaints were allowed to be admitted to the study. This had led to a relatively young study population, which then offered an ideal situation to study typical climacteric complaints. The drop-out pattern did not differ between the two treatment groups. (Breslow test > 0.05).

Results

Hot flushes were effectively reduced with both preparations. It was generally observed that oral substitution needs at least 3 to 4 treatment cycles, until the highest possible success rates are achieved (Fig. 2). Therefore, physicians should encourage the patient to continue therapy for a certain period, instead of immediately switching to higher estrogen dosages.

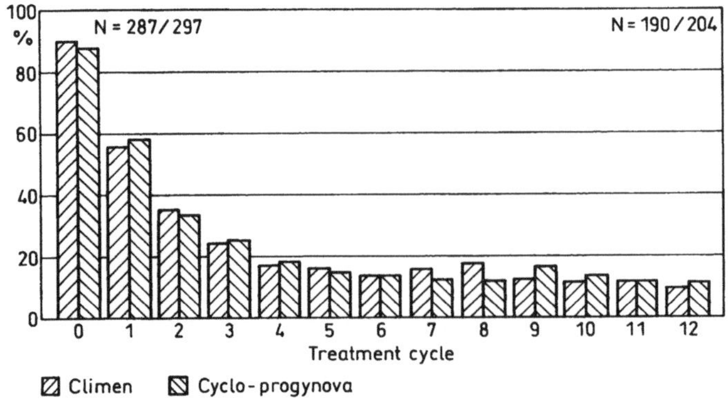

Fig. 2: Effects on hot flushes

Table 1: Study population (Clinical study SH D 461 AZ/83001)

Age	%
less than 45 years	20.4
45–49 years	35.0
50–54 years	28.8
55 years and more	15.8
Menopausal status	
Premenopause	44.8
Postmenopause	45.2
Duration of complaints	
less than 6 months	25.6
7–12 months	24.1
1–3 years	24.6
more than 3 years	25.8

As we had seen many patients with severe forms of vasomotoric complaints, so was their sleep pattern frequently disturbed. Before starting treatment, 60% complained of insomnia. In particular those, who suffered badly from insomnia reported a resumption or at least an amelioration of their normal sleep pattern. The same can be said for the treatment group with Cyclo-Progynova (Fig. 3).

Approximately 60% of the patients reported depressive changes of mood. Three quarters of these women reported a relief of these complaints after 12 treatment cycles.

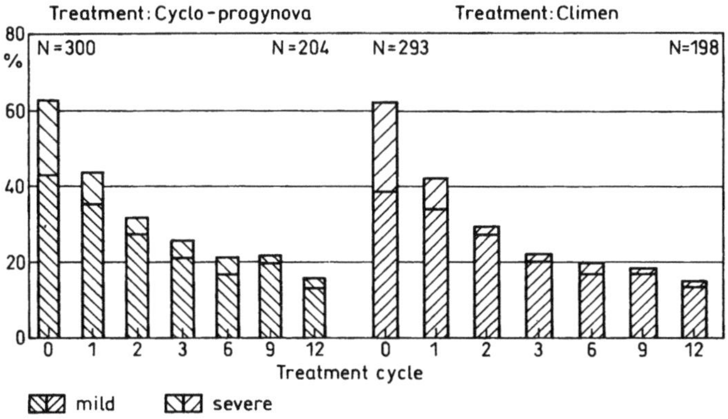

Fig. 3: Effects on insomnia

If moderate forms of depression coincide with pronounced vasomotoric instability, HRT is very likely to contribute to a psychic stabilisation. This effect is supported by the present result. One may assume that androgenic and antiandrogenic progestins have different influences on the psyche. However, the results of this study did not reveal any differences between the two treatment groups in this respect.

Estrogen deficiency leads to an atrophy of hormone-dependent tissue of the urogenital tract. This may cause a number of secondary diseases, e. g. problems of incontinence or frequency of urogenital infections. Symptoms related to urogenital atrophy were present in one quarter of the study population. These symptoms ameliorated or disappeared in the course of both treatments.

Our results confirm, that headache is a common complaint of the climacteric period. On the other hand, headaches may also appear as a side-effect of hormonal therapy. However, the net result of the influence of HRT in our study shows that the percentage of patients with headaches is reduced by half following both treatments. Most patients who continued to experience headache also during therapy reported the symptom to be either improved or unchanged under both therapies. Therefore, it appears, as both preparations show the same pattern, the progestational compound obviously does not seem to influence the incidence of headaches.

When estrogen production by the ovaries ceases, adrenal androgenes become more dominant. Susceptible patients may perceive skin changes like seborrhoea and acne. Severe forms may even result in hirsutism. With 1 mg cyproterone acetate, one cannot expect a real contribution via its antiandrogenic properties. But what about the 19-nor-testosterone derivative norgestrel? Following Climen, a trend towards a lower percentage of patients with acne could be observed as compared to Cyclo-Progynova, although not statistically significant. Baseline values were higher in the Climen group (Fig. 4).

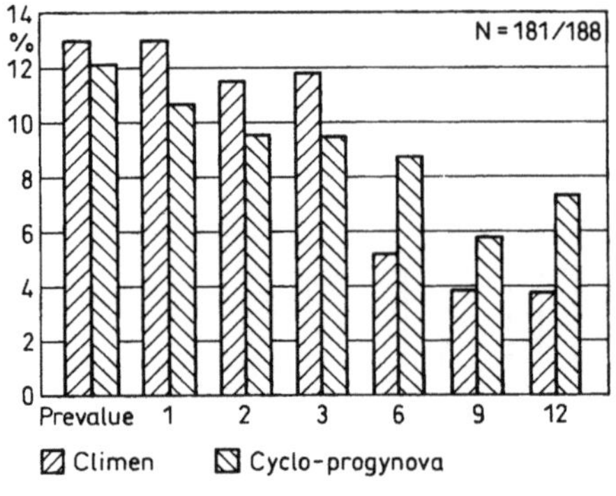

Fig. 4: Effects on acne

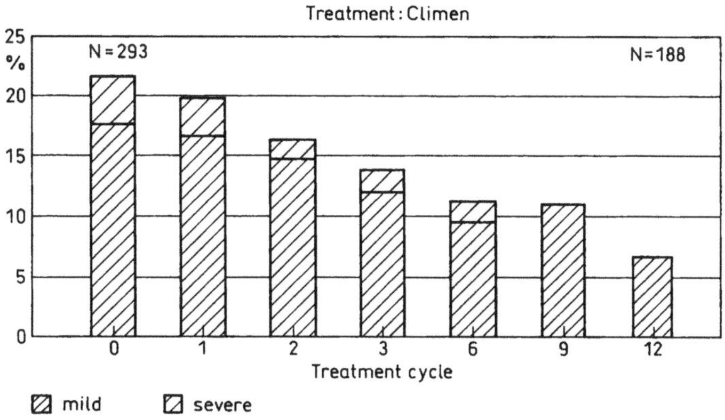

Fig. 5: Effects on seborrhoea

The percentage of patients reporting seborrhea in the Climen group declined with prolonged treatment; none of the patients classified the symptom as severe in the 9th or 12th cycle (Fig. 5).

Both treatments caused regular withdrawal bleedings in about 80–90% of all cycles; amenorrhea was reported somewhat more frequently in the Climen group. Cyclo-Progynova produced a more favourable cycle stability reflected in the lower incidence of spotting.

Irregular menstruation-like bleeding and spotting occurred more frequently in young premenopausal women. There were less irregular bleedings in women after the menopause in both treatment groups.

While treated, more than 70% of the patients kept their body weight constant and increased it by more than 2 kg in only 20% (Fig. 6). There was no difference between treatment groups (Cyclo-Progynova in study 83001 and Trisequens in study 83121).

There was no significant change in systolic blood pressure after 12 treatment cycles in comparison to baseline values in both treatment groups. However, only in the Climen-group were there more decreases than increases in systolic blood pressure. The same holds true for diastolic blood pressure. The following laboratory results have been published by Hirvonen et. al [1]. HDL-cholesterol is often regarded as a protective factor for coronary heart disease. Treatment with Climen did not influence HDL-cholesterol values, in contrast to Cyclo-Progynova where HDL-cholesterol was lowered after the third treatment month (Fig. 7). HRT with Climen leads to a decrease of LDL-cholesterol plasma levels, which was statistically significant ($p < 0.05$). The LDL-cholesterol low-

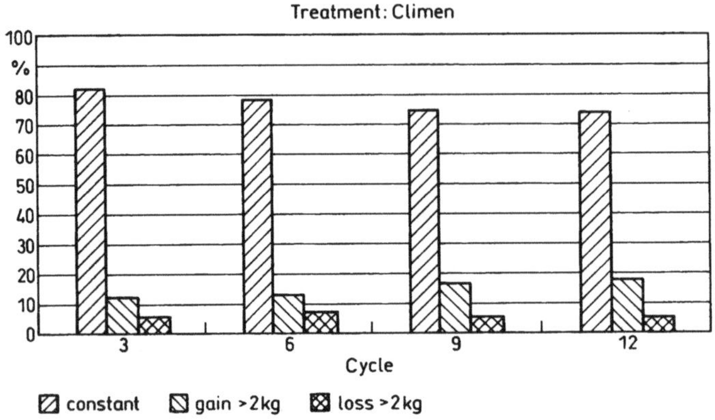

Fig. 6: Effects on body weight

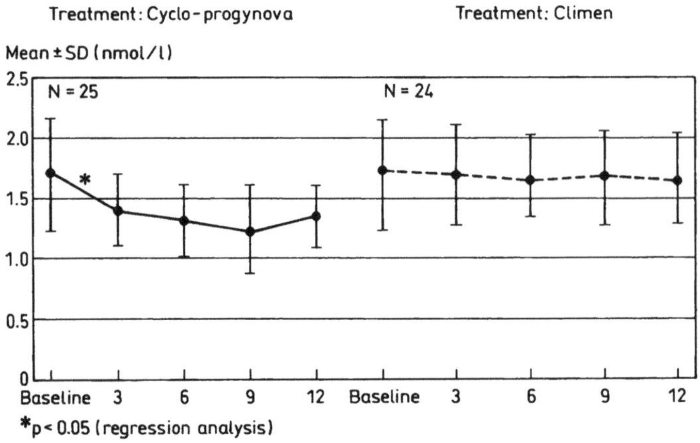

Fig. 7: Effects on HDL-cholesterol

ering effect of 2 mg estradiol valerate could also be demonstrated in the treatment group with Cyclo-Progynova (regression analysis revealed a decrease; $p < 0.05$, Fig. 8).

Changes in the lipoprotein pattern confirmed our theoretical considerations. LDL-C appeared to have decreased under therapy with both regimens ($p < 0.05$). However, norgestrel lowered HDL-C concomitantly. This result showed an impairment of the atherogenic index which dropped from 0.36 to 0.32. In contrast, HDL-C levels under CPA remained constant. As a result the atherogenic index improved by rising from 0.38 to 0.43 on average.

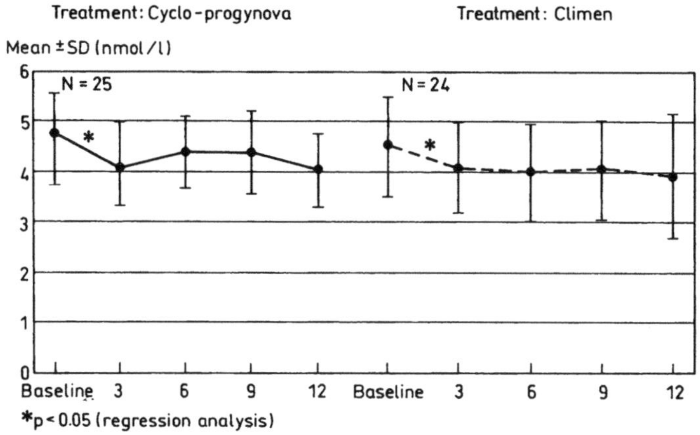

Fig. 8: Effects on LDL-cholesterol

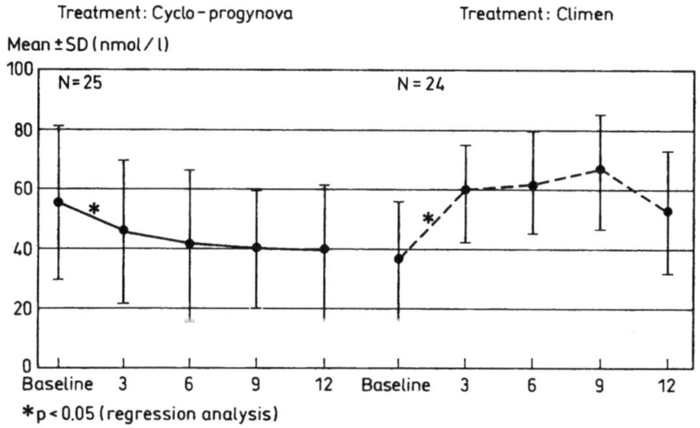

Fig. 9: Effects on sex-hormone-binding globuline (SHBG)

Estrogens are known to induce SHBG synthesis in the liver. This effect could also be demonstrated under Climen (Fig. 9). The increase of SHBG plasma levels was statistically significant ($p < 0.05$).

With Cyclo-Progynova, the induction of SHBG synthesis in the liver is counteracted by the androgenic progestin norgestrel ($p < 0.05$). Changes of SHBG values under therapy demonstrated likewise the different origin of norgestrel and CPA. Whereas norgestrel produced a decrease of SHBG plasma levels, CPA produced an increase ($p < 0.05$). Hence, as liver protein synthesis is stimulated by estrogens, the latter regimen has a more estrogenic profile.

Conclusion

A sequential regimen with estradiol valerate (2 mg) and the addition of a progestational compound is able to reduce climacteric complaints. This study demonstrates that the type of progestogen does not influence this therapeutic benefit. A comparison of both estradiol valerate and conjugated estrogens is pinpointed in Table 2 which would favour the natural estradiol for replacement.

Table 2: Comparison of conjugated estrogens and estradiol valerate

Conjugated estrogens	Estradiol valerate
Metabolism and pharmacokinetics of the different components of conjugated estrogens not fully known	Prodrug of 17β-estradiol, a human estrogen
More pronounced effect on synthesis of hepatic serum proteins	

Both preparations were equally effective in reducing climacteric complaints. As with other oral treatment regimens, symptom relief can be expected within some 3–4 treatment cycles. Together with the reduction of vasomotoric complaints, other less specific complaints may improve, e. g. insomnia, depression, headaches. Only a few patients experience headaches as a side-effect of the hormone substitution.

Laboratory investigations confirmed the hypothesis that progestins from the class of 19-nor-testosterone are able to counteract the estrogen-induced changes in lipoprotein pattern. Even though LDL-C levels were found to be reduced under therapy with either of the preparations, the decrease was more pronounced with CPA. Moreover the HDL-C levels remained unchanged with the CPA-containing preparation, while it was decreased under norgestrel. In consequence, the atherogenic index was more favourably influenced by CPA than norgestrel.

Skin changes, attributable to an androgenic influence, may also improve. Cyclo-Progynova appears to intensify problems of seborrhoea via its androgenic progestin.

Discussion

Both preparations proved to be effective in reducing typical climacteric complaints. The regimens led to monthly withdrawal bleedings in most patients.

The probable pattern of bleeding depends greatly on the particular estrogen/progestogen regimen but also on the individual responsiveness among the women treated. Women who have bled erratically during the intake of one preparation are more likely to have the same problems with irregular bleedings under HRT than premenopausal women.

In recent years, sequential estrogen-progestogen regimens have constituted the standard approach to long-term postmenopausal hormone replacement therapy. This virtually eliminates the risk of endometrial hyperplasia and carcinoma. Bleeding patterns with these regimens are more predictable than with others, but are certainly not perfect.

The duration of progestogen addition rather than the daily dosages, appears to be the crucial factor for reducing the incidence of hyperplasia. To recall the important figures, estrogen monotherapy leads to hyperplasia in approximately 20–30%. An addition of progestogen for 7 days reduces the incidence to 4% and with 10–12 days of this addition, the occurrence of endometrial hyperplasia is reduced to almost zero.

The excellent cycle stability under 0.5 mg norgestrel is not surprising as this dosage is very high. It equals 0.25 mg of levonorgestrel, and we know that even one fourth of this dosage would be sufficient to protect the endometrium from overstimulation.

Thus, by increasing the progestogen dosage beyond the threshold of preventing endometrial hyperplasia, one may be able to reduce the rate of irregular bleedings to a certain extent. There is, however, doubt about the metabolic hazard of high dosages of progestogens, especially when they have androgenic properties.

Patients who tend to have heavy irregular bleedings under HRT will certainly benefit from the norgestrel containing preparation. Under the assumption that for irregular bleedings organic reasons are excluded, it may be administered for a short-term intervention. For a long-term treatment, however, the CPA-containing preparation should be preferred.

CPA proved its neutral behaviour with respect to lipoprotein pattern. This must be concluded out of clinical studies, published by Tikkanen, Hirvonen, Christiansen and others. Furthermore, the Danish research group of Christiansen was able to demonstrate a bone conserving effect of the 2 mg EV + 1 mg CPA preparation [3]. Thus, it may be an excellent preparation for treatment of the climacteric syndrome and for prevention of postmenopausal osteoporosis and possibly cardiovascular diseases.

References

[1] Hirvonen, E., J. Elliesen, K. Schmidt-Gollwitzer: Comparison of two hormone replacement regimens – influence on lipoproteins and bone mineral content. Maturitas *12* (1990) 127–136.

[2] Ottosson, U. B., B. G. Johansson, B. von Schoultz: Subfractions of high-density lipoprotein cholesterol during estrogen replacement therapy: a comparison between progestogen and natural progesterone. Am. J. Obstet. Gynecol. *151* (1985) 746–750.

[3] Riis, B. J., J. Jensen, C. Christiansen: Cyproterone acetate, an alternative gestagen in postmenopausal oestrogen/gestagen therapy. Clin. Endocrinol. *26* (1987) 327–334.

[4] Tikkanen, M. J., T. Kuusi, E. A. Nikkilä et al.: Post-heparin plasma hepatic lipase activity as a predictor of high-density lipoprotein response to progestogen therapy: studies with cyproterone acetate. Maturitas *9* (1987) 81–86.

Cyproterone acetate as progestin in the treatment of climacteric disorders

A. R. Genazzani, F. Petraglia, N. Mercuri, A. D. Genazzani, M. R. Sgherzi, L. Aguzzoli, C. Volpogni

Introduction

The lack of menstruation is the critical event that heralds a new era in a woman's progression through life. A more accurate term for this time of transition is the 'climacteric' (42–54 years of age), since this includes the premenopausal and postmenopausal periods. It is mainly characterized by events resulting from the estrogen deficit.

The climacteric syndrome

The climacteric syndrome is the combination of various short- and long-term symptoms. The short-term consequences are represented by vasomotoric instability (hot flushes, night sweats), neurogenic disturbances (depression, anxiety, migrainoid headaches, insomnia), skin collagen loss, lipidaemia, atrophic vaginits, urinary incontinence and nocturia unaccounted for by anatomical change, bacterial infection of urogenital tract, all symptoms associated with hormonal imbalance. The long-term consequence is represented by the osteoporosis that derives from the postmenopausal bone loss. For women undergoing menopause around 50 years of age, prospective studies have shown a continous decrease in radial and vertebral bone mass from this time and an increased incidence of osteoporotic fractures.

The estrogen replacement treatment (ERT) is the optimal approach to solve the symptoms of the climacteric syndrome. However, a progestin must be associated to the estrogens in planning a substitutive treatment. A wide spectrum of biological action of progestins has been elucidated by a large number of experimental and clinical implications (Fig. 1).

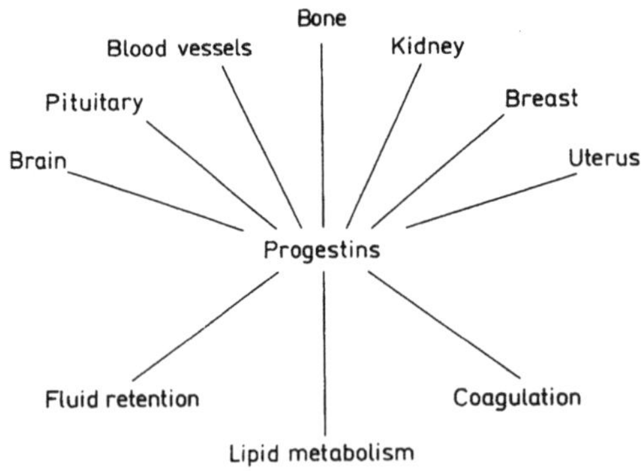

Fig. 1: Progestins have several target organs with multiple implications in human physiology

Biological actions of progestins

Progestins and endometrium

Since the first retrospective studies indicated that the risk of endometrial carcinoma from estrogen replacement therapy (ERT) [19–32] was increased three to ten-fold, a 10–13 day course of progestagens has been advocated for routine use with estrogen therapy [11–28] given their preventive effect on endometrial hyperplasia.

It has been shown that progesterone stimulates endometrial 17-B-dehydrogenase activity, leading to an accelerated conversion of estradiol (E2) to estrone (E1) [26]. This effect has a direct relevance to the antiestrogenicity of progesterone and progestins and the net result is a lowering of the endometrial concentration of E2. Progesterone and progestins decrease estrogen receptor levels in the endometrium [26], probably in inhibiting the rate of synthesis of the estrogen receptors. The final result is that progesterone inhibits ephitelial cell growth and multiplication, stimulating cell differentiation, and slowing down the cell cycle process [18].

Progestins and breast

In human breast tissue the progestins are able to increase the progesterone (P) receptor concentration in the nucleus [16]. The 17-B-hydroxysteroid dehydrogenase activity (E2DH) can be considered to be the marker of P receptor activity, leading to the conversion of estradiol to estrone [26, 10, 29]. Then, in breast tissue, just as in the endometrium, progesterone and progestins exert an antiestrogenic activity through both mechanisms: decrease in E2 receptors and increase in E2DH activity, leading to lower E2 concentrations in the target tissue. However, recent findings have shown that progestins may have an effect on cell proliferation [3].

Progestins and brain

Progesterone receptors have been found in the central nervous system in animals [21]. Progesterone itself exerts hypnotic effects through its 3a-reduced metabolites and has been referred to as effective in relieving premenstrual anxiety and psychological disability [7], thus confirming an action of progesterone on the central nervous system, as was previously suggested [1]. Moreover, when a massive increase in plasma progesterone occurs, psychological complaints recorded are of sedation sometimes associated with drowsiness.

Progesterone and progestins have the capacity to modify the neurohormone and neuropeptide contents in the brain. The neuroendocrine change following ovariectomy may be influenced by the administration of progesterone or progestins.

In particular, ovariectomy increases gonadotropin-releasing-hormone (GnRH) in the hypothalamus of rats and the chronic administration of progesterone or norethisterone enanthate (NET) further increases such levels [14]. Moreover, progesterone and NET counteract the estradiol-induced GnRH decrease [14]. No changes have been shown following desogestrel or medroxyprogesterone acetate (MAP) treatment.

The influence on GnRH contents reflects the capacity of progesterone and progestins to modulate the hypothalamic-pituitary-gonadal axis. The different activity of the various progestins indicate that these molecules have different capacities to bind to the progesterone receptors within the hypothalamus.

Different effects of progesterone and progestin have also been shown on brain beta-endorphin contents. It is well known that beta-endorphin and the opioid peptides play several and relevant roles in the central nervous system (Fig. 2). Mood, sexual behavior, feeding behavior, pain perception, and neuroendocrine regulation of the pituitary-ovarian axis have been shown for brain beta-endorphin [12]. In ovariectomized rats hypothalamic beta-endorphin decreases after 3–5 weeks from surgery [24]. The administration of progesterone, NET or norgestimate is able to increase beta-endorphin contents above the control values, while MAP or desogestrel have no effects [13, 15].

Therefore, a differential action of progestins is clearly shown on the hypothalamic neurons. In agreement with this conclusion other reports have shown that cyproterone acetate (CPA) chronically administered to ovariectomized rats

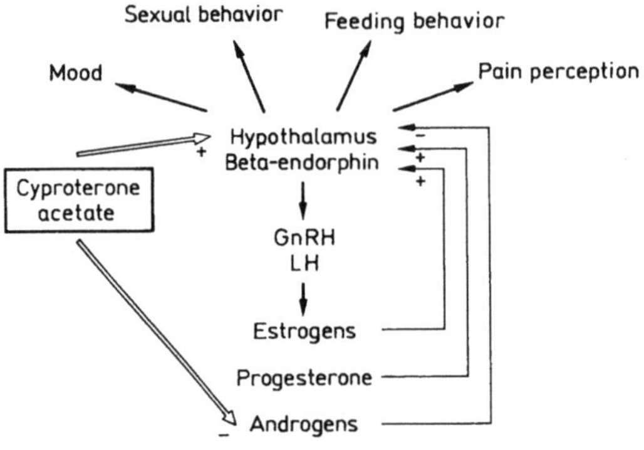

Fig. 2: The steroid hormone beta-endorphin pathway is one of the central targets of cyproterone acetate

increases beta-endorphin contents in the hypothalamus (Fig. 2) [15]. The effect of CPA was dose-dependent [15]. Furthermore, CPA enhances the estrogen effect and counteracts the androgen inhibitor on hypothalamic beta-endorphin [15]. The positive effect of CPA is also evident on anterior and intermediate lobe pituitary gland beta-endorphin contents. The different activity of these progestins on the brain neuropeptides may explain the different effects of the various gestagens on mood changes and psychologic symptom relief typical of the HRT in postmenopausal women. In view of the failure to antagonize the estrogen central effect, CPA seems of particular interest as progestin for postmenopausal complains.

Progestins and bone

While the preventive treatment of estrogens on osteoporosis is well known, the role of progestogens is still in doubt since the mechanism of action of progestogens on the skeleton is yet unclear. Human and animal experiments give conflicting results, some suggesting reduced turnover, others failing to detect this.

Probably, progestogens could interact with glucocorticoid receptors in bone, but it is not clear whether the interaction is evident in physiological conditions or under pharmacological concentrations of progestogen treatment [20]. Norethisterone reduces bone loss without any effect on urinary hydroxyproline [20]. However, from these studies, it appears to be clear that the addition of progesterone to estrogen does not play a major role in the action of estrogen in the prevention of bone loss in postmenopausal therapy.

Progestins and metabolism

The effect of progesterone and its derivates have been shown to exert minimal changes on lipid profiles. The 19-nortestosterone derivatives with androgenic properties are known to stimulate hepatic lipoprotein lipase (HL) and decrease liver synthesis of high density lipoproteins (HDL) with a concomitant increase in low density lipoprotein (LDL) [5]. Low levels of HDL and/or high levels of LDL are in theory associated with excess storage of cholesterol (C) in the vascular walls and subsequent development of atherosclerosis and related cardiovascular disease (CVD) [17]. It has been shown that some progestins (NET, norgestrel) interpose in the intrahepatic cholesterol metabolism, reducing HDL and increasing LDL-cholesterol fractions, while a new generation of 19-norprogesterones (desogestrel, norgestimate, gestoden) have no effect and CPA, for its antiandrogenic properties, clearly shows its favourable effect inducing an antiatherogenic profile of plasma lipids. These considerations must be of even greater relevance in the treatment of estrogen-deficiency symptoms, because women in the age group concerned suffer a much higher incidence of CVD than younger women.

Concerning the role progestins play on coagulation no modification of antithrombin III (AT III) with chlormadione acetate, retrogesterone, ethynodiol diacetate or norgestrienone was observed [23]. In postmenopausal women receiving oral micronized progesterone, no changes in platelet aggregation, factor VII, AT III or fibrinolytic capacity were found [22].

It has been shown that changes in the renin-aldosterone system occurred under various progestins. Progesterone exerts an antimineralcorticoid effect, by competing with aldosterone for binding with its receptors [27] and a natriuretic effect [22], while some progestogens cause slight sodium retention [2, 31].

Moreover, estrogen and progesterone exhibit an antagonist action on vascular permeability [6, 30] and increasing doses of progestins in estrogen-treated animals lower the vascular permeability and fluid retention [6].

Cyproterone acetate as progestin for treating the climacteric syndrome

Cyproterone acetate has many positive biological effects and less side-effects. In particular, the increases of HDL-C and the concomitant decreases of LDL-C induced by a chronic treatment with CPA (combined with estrogen) is one of the clinical advantages.

Starting from the concept that progestin, in association with the unopposed estrogen therapy, is used for the treatment of women in their postmenopause with the sole purpose of protecting them from endometrial hyperplasia and cancer, several observations concerning the selection of the most adequate molecule can be made for reasons of safety and efficacy.

In this context, the positive antiandrogenic effect of CPA on skin and other androgen-sensitive epidermal structures antagonizes the adrenal androgen activity at this level, improving the general feminine aspect of the treated women. The positive activity on lipid fractions reduces the cardiovascular risks and increases the great protection associated with the HRT. The positive effect of CPA on central and peripheral opioids counteracts this typical biochemical symptom of menopause and seems to play a major role in the improvement of physical symptoms associated with the climacteric syndrome.

References

[1] Backstrom, T., A. Cartensen: Estrogen and progesterone in plasma in relation to premenstrual tension. J. Steroid. Biochem. *5* (1974) 257–260.

[2] Cecil, H. C., J. A. Hannun, J. Bitman: Quantitative characterization of uterine permeability changes with estrogen. Am. J. Physiol. *211* (1966) 1099–1102.

[3] Christine, L., C. Sutherland, R. L. Sutherland: Progestin regulation of cellular proliferation. End. Rev. *11* (1990) 266.

[4] Conrad, J., M. Samama, M. H. Horellao et al.: Antithrombin III and oral contraceptive with prostagen-only preparation. Lancet *II* (1979) 41.

[5] Crona, N., L. Enk, L. A. Mattson et al.: Progestogens and lipid metabolism. Maturitas *8* (1986) 91–176.

[6] Das Gupta, P. R., M. Ghost, J. R. Pande et al.: Anti-estrogenicity of norgestrel. Current Sci. *20* (1970) 467–468.

[7] Dennerstein, L., C. Spencer-Gardener, G. Gotts et al.: Progesterone and the premenstrual syndrome: a double blind crossover trial. Br. Med. J. *290* (1985) 1617–1621.

[8] De Wied, D., Tj. B. van Wimersma Greidaus: The neuropeptide concept and the menopause. In: L. Zichella, M. I. Whitehead, P. A. van Keep (eds.): The climacteric and beyond, pp. 3–18. The Parthenon Publishing Group Ltd., Carnforth 1987.

[9] Fahraeus, L., U. Larsson-Cohn, L. Wallentin: Norgestrel and progesterone have different influences on plasma lipoproteins. Eur. J. Clin. Invest. *13* (1983) 447–453.

[10] Fournier, S., F. Kutten, F. de Cicco et al.: Estradriol 17-B-hydroxysteroid dehydrogenase activity in human breast fibroadenomas. J. Clin. Endocrinol. Metab. *55* (1982) 428–433.

[11] Gambrell, D. R. jr.: Prevention of endometrial cancer with progestogens. Maturitas *8* (1986) 159–168.

[12] Genazzani, A. R., F. Petraglia, M. Bergamaschi et al.: Progesterone and progestins modulate B-endorphin concentrations in the hypothalamus and the pituitary of castrated female rats. Gynecol. Endocrinol. *1* (1987) 61 – 69.

[13] Genazzani, A. R., F. Petraglia, M. Cleva et al.: Norgestimate increases pituitary and hypothalamic concentrations of immunoreactive beta-endorphin. Contracept. *5* (1989) 605 – 613.

[14] Genazzani, A. R., F. Petraglia, M. Silferi et al.: Progestins modulate the action of estrogen on gonadotropin-releasing hormone, luteinizing hormone, and prolactin in the rat. Gynecol. Obstet. Invest. *29* (1990) 197 – 202.

[15] Genazzani, A. R., F. Petraglia, N. Mercuri et al.: Effect of steroid hormones and antihormones on hypothalamic beta-endorphin concentrations in intact and castrated female rats. J. Endocrinol. Invest. *13* (1990) 91 – 96.

[16] Gerchenson, L. E., C. Conner, J. T. Murai: Regulation of cell cycle by diethylstilbestrol and progesterone in cultured endometrial cells. Endocrinol. *100* (1977) 1468 – 1471.

[17] Gordon, T., W. P. Castelli, M. C. Hjortland et al.: High density lipoprotein as a protective factor against coronary heart disease. Am. J. Med. *62* (1977) 707 – 714.

[18] Hsueh, A. J. W., E. J. Peck, J. H. Clark: Central of uterine estrogen receptor levels by progesterone. Endocrinol. *98* (1976) 438 – 444.

[19] Jick, H., R. N. Watkins, J. R. Hunter et al.: Replacement estrogens and endometrial cancer. N. Engl. J. Med. *300* (1979) 218 – 222.

[20] Lindsay, R.: Oral communication. IVth International Congress of the Menopause, Lake Buena Vista, Florida, U. S. A. 1984.

[21] MacLusky, N. J., B. S. MacEwen: Progestin receptors in the brain and pituitary of the bonnet monkey: differences between the monkey and the rat in the distribution of progestin receptors. Endocrinol. *106* (1980) 185 – 191.

[22] Oelkers, W., M. Schoneshofer, A. Blumel: Effect of progesterone and four synthetic progestogens on sodium balance and the renin aldosterone in man. J. Clin. Endocrinol. Metab. *39* (1974) 882 – 890.

[23] Sitruk-Ware, R., C. Bricaire, B. De Lignieres et al.: Oral micronized progesterone. A review. Contraception *36* (1987) 373 – 402.

[24] Petraglia, F., A. Penalva, V. Locatelli et al.: Effect of gonadectomy and gonadal steroid replacement on pituitary and plasma B-endorphin levels in the rats. Endocrinol. *111* (1982) 1224.

[25] Tikkanen, M. J., E. A. Nikkila, E. A. Kuusi: Reduction of plasma high-density lipoprotein 2 cholesterol and increase of postheparin plasma hepatic lipase activity during progestin treatment. Clin. Chim. Acta *115* (1981) 63 – 71.

[26] Tseng, L., E. Gurpide: Induction of human endometrial estradiol dehydrogenase by progestins. Endocrinol. *98* (1976) 438 – 444.

[27] Wambach, G., J. R. Higgins, D. C. L. Kem.: Interaction of synthetic progestogens with renal mineralcorticoid receptors. Acta Endocrinol. *92* (1979) 560 – 567.

[28] Whitehead, M. I.: The effects of estrogens and progestagens on the postmenopausal endometrium. Maturitas *1* (1978) 87 – 98.

[29] Whitehead, M. I., P. T. Townsend, J. Pryse – Davis: Effects of estrogens and progestins on the biochemistry and morphology of the postmenopausal endometrium. N. Engl. J. Med. *305* (1981) 1599 – 1605.

[30] Whitehead, M. I., P. T. Townsend, D. K. Gillet et al.: Absorption and metabolism of oral progesterone. Br. Med. J. *280* (1980) 825–827.

[31] Zeppa, R.: Vascular response of breast to estrogen. J. Clin. Endocrinol. Metab. *29* (1969) 695–701.

[32] Ziel, H. K., W. C. Finkle: Increased risk of endometrial carcinoma among users of conjugated estrogens. N. Engl. J. Med. *293* (1975) 1167–1170

The effects of a sequential estradiol-valerate cyproterone acetate preparation on the endometrium during hormone replacement therapy

P. R. Koninckx, J. A. Lauweryns, F. J. Cornillie

Abstract

Three sequential estradiol valerate (EV) cyproterone acetate (CPA) combination products with 11 days of estrogen and 10 days of estrogen and progestagen were investigated during hormone replacement therapy in 2 prospective double-blind randomised trials. SH D A contained 2 mg of EV and 1 mg of CPA, SH D B 1 mg and 0.5 mg and SH D G 2 mg and 2 mg respectively.

During SH D A treatment, hot flushes ($P < 0.0001$), night sweats ($P < 0.0001$), depression ($P = 0.0001$), dizziness ($P = 0.0001$) and insomnia ($P = 0.003$) decreased significantly. No side-effects occurred except breast tenderness in 18% of women. Weight, blood pressure, thyroid function, adrenal function, liver function, kidney function, parathyroid hormone and vitamin D, platelets and blood cell count did not change during 12 months of therapy.

Women treated with SH D A had mestruations, which decreased in volume during the first months of treatment ($P < 0.0001$), being scanty in $\pm$ 30%, whereas $\pm$ 10% had amenorrhea. Spotting occurred in $\pm$ 10%. The endometrial biopsy was athrophic in 5–10% of women, showed a perfectly normal secretory phase in 45%, and irregular secretion in 45% of women. After careful analysis, using visual analog scales this was interpreted as a strong progestagenic effect; women treated with SH D A had, in comparison with normal menstrual cycles, a more heterogenic glandular epithelium with more papillae, larger stromal cells, a more pronounced decidual reaction and more fibrinoid material. Hyperplasia was not seen in any woman.

SH D B in comparison with SH D A was less effective for the treatment of menopausal complaints. Amenorrhea occurred in 50%, but irregular bleedings were troublesome in over 20%. The endometrial biopsy was athropic in 57%.

SH D G in comparison with SH D A was equally effective in treating flushes, sweats, dizziness, and depression. Also the decrease in menstrual flow during the first months, the $\pm$ 10% amenorrhea and the $\pm$ 10% atrophic endometria were comparable. The detailed analysis revealed an even stronger progestagenic effect than in SH D A.

In conclusion: SH D A is the product of choice in comparison with SH D B and SH D G. It is highly effective in treating menopausal complaints, has no side effects except breast tenderness, has good cycle control and induces a physiologic secretory transformation in the endometrium. The dose of 1 mg CPA is high normal progestagenic, which can be considered an advantage for the prevention of endometrial hyperplasia.

Introduction

The benefits of hormone replacement therapy have become widely recognised over the last decade; postmenopausal vasomotor symptoms and atrophy are effectively treated, osteoporosis can be prevented and the risk of cardiovascular accidents is probably decreased [3, 5, 14].

The risk and prevention of endometrial hyperplasia is, however, still a major concern. Progestagens are therefore recommended to be given monthly for at least 10 days [3, 16] in order to prevent endometrial hyperplasia, to induce a more regular desquamation and ultimately to prevent endometrial malignant transformation.

The effect of progestagens upon the endometrium is mediated through a decrease of estrogen receptors [10], an increase of the 17α-oxydoreductase activity converting estradiol to estrone [11]. They inhibit endometrial mitotic activity as evidenced by a decrease in the number of mitoses [8, 9], both in the glandular epithelium and in the stroma and they induce the well-known secretory transformations. Although these effects are clearly dose-related [18], the exact dose-effects-relationships remain largely unknown because of an important interindividual variability [13] complex estroprogestagen interactions [6] and the absence of a useful animal model. For most synthetic progestagens only the minimal effective doses to prevent endometrial hyperplasia have been investigated in the human [13, 18].

Since a careful morphometric analysis of large numbers of endometrial biopsies would represent an enormous and almost impossible task, whereas descriptive data are difficult to analyse statistically, a semi-quantitative method using visual analog scales has been developed to evaluate secretory transformation in endometrial biopsies and this method was used to evaluate sequential estro-progestagen hormone replacement products containing cyproterone acetate as a progestagen.

Materials and methods

Treatments

The treatments given in this study consisted of 11 days of estradiol valerate (EV), 10 days of the same dose of estradiol valerate together with cyproterone acetate (CPA) followed by a 7 day tablet free interval. Three drug regimens were used: SH D A contained 2 mg EV and 1 mg CPA, SH D B 1 mg EV and 0.5 mg CPA and SH D G 2 mg EV and 2 mg CPA.

Study design

The first study was a prospective randomised double-blind trial of SH D A and SH D B in 40 postmenopausal women for 6 months, followed by an open period of 9 months. The second study was a prospective randomised double-blind trial of SH D A and SH D G in 30 women for 4 months.

Menopausal symptoms, bleeding and side-effects were recorded daily by the patient for 1 month before therapy and during therapy and by the physician at the monthly or 2 monthly follow up visits. Flushes and night sweats were recorded as frequent when they occurred more than 5 times/day or 3 times/night and as severe when abundant sweating and discomfort was present. Fasting blood samples and endometrial biopsies were taken before therapy and during the last week of tablet intake.

Patients

All women were seen at the menopause clinic of the University Hospital Gasthuisberg for menopausal complaints. The inclusion criteria were a natural menopause since more than 6 months, an intact uterus, the absence of any hormonal treatment for at least 3 months, and a written informal consent by the patient. Exclusion criteria were severe liver function disturbances, jaundice or general pruritus during a previous pregnancy, Dubin Johnson's Syndrome, Rotor Syndrome, a previous thromboembolic process, sickle-cell anaemia, history of or existing breast carcinoma or adenocarcinoma of the endometrium or other possibly hormone-dependent tumors, congenital disturbances of lipid metabolism, otosclerosis with deterioration in a previous pregnancy or a history of herpes gestationis during pregnancy. In both studies the women enrolled were comparable for age, weight, height and duration of menopause, incidence of previous therapy and smoking (Tab. 1).

Table 1: Patient characteristics

	Study I		Study II	
	SH D B	SH D A	SH D A	SH D G
n	20	20	15	15
Height (cm)	164 ± 8	161 ± 6	161 ± 6	162 ± 7
Age (years)	48 ± 8	46 ± 9	49 ± 4	51 ± 5
Duration of menopause				
< 1 year (%)	47	38	91	77
> 3 years (%)	13	15	7	11
No previous therapy (%)	61	56	73	67
Smoker (%)	18	21	20	20

Endometrial biopsies

Endometrial biopsies were taken with a Novak curette, fixed in acetaldehyde formaldehyde (study I) or in Bouin (study II), imbedded in epon or paraffin, and stained with toluidine blue or hematoxylin-eosin respectively. Endometrial biopsies were evaluated carefully at the Department of Pathology for any signs of hyperplasia, adenomatous hyperplasia, or malignant transformation, and dated blindly according to the criteria of Noyes et al. [2, 15]. Moreover all biopsies were scored blindly on a visual analog scale (Fig. 1). This method was validated by scoring blindly endometrial biopsies taken in women with a regular cycle, and a duration of the luteal phase between 12 and 16 days. In these women the exact day of the luteal phase was established in relationship with the LH peak (n = 71) or the basal body temperature rise (n = 60) for endometrial biopsies taken between day 14 and 22 of the mentrual cycle, or with the onset of menstruation (n = 51) for endometrial biopsies taken between day 20 and 28 of the menstrual cycle. The day of LH-peak and menstruation were considered as day 13 and 28 respectively. Since most of these women were investigated for infertility only biopsies which by dating were less than 3 days out of phase were used, in order to eliminate luteal phase insufficiencies. In order to avoid premature bleeding in cycles in which the endometrial biopsy had been taken, women with a plasma progesterone concentration higher than 2 ng/ml were not included in the control series which consisted of 16 biopsies taken before day 10, 19 taken day 10–14, 17 day 15–16, 18 day 17–18, 30 day 19–20, 17 day 21–22, 12 day 23–24, 18 day 25–26 and 5 day 27–28 respectively. In women taking SH D A, SH D B or SH D G, the first day of tablet intake containing CPA was considered day 14.

ENDOMETRIAL BIOPSY		
BIOPSY	Insufficient — Sufficient	
Height		
% Epith/Stroma		100% str
Gland Dilat		+++
EPITHELIUM		
Homogeneity		no
Height		Cylindr
Pseudostrat		+++
Mitoses		5/10 ×
Papil		+++
Basal Vacuol		+++
Intralum Secr		+++
STROMA		
Nucl/Cytopl		
Mitoses		5/10 ×
Edema		+++
Capill		+++
		dilated
K-cel		+++
Foam-cel		+++
Spiral arter		+++
Predecid		+++
CONCLUSION		
Hyperpl		GCH
Adenom Hyperpl		clear
Secretion		normal

Fig. 1: Visual analog scales used to assess endometrial histology.

Assays

Luteinising hormone (LH), Follicle stimulating hormone (FSH) and progesterone were assayed using the Medgenix kits (Medgenix, 6220 Fleurus, Belgium). Prolactin (PRL), progesterone, 17β-estradiol (E_2), estrone (E_1), testosterone, parathyroid hormone, vitamin D, cortisol, transcortin and sex-hormone-binding-globulin (SHBG) were assayed as described previously [1, 7, 12]; thyroid hormones were determined by the Abbott kit, and blood biochemistry was done on a SMAC auto-analyser.

Data analysis

Data analysis was performed using the SAS package [17], and statistical significance was evaluated using Students t-test, chi-square test and analysis of variance (the GLM procedure was used for analysis of variance with unequal cell sizes). Unless stated otherwise means $\pm$ SD or mean (25th-75th percentile) are given for normally and skewed distributions respectively.

Results

Patients acceptance and drop outs

In the first study 17 out of 20 women finished the six month SH D A trial. One woman stopped treatment after one month because of insufficient relief of symptoms and an imminent trip to the middle east, whereas two preferred to use another preparation with a higher dosage, which they had been using 4 months previously. Treatment B was continued in 15 out of 20 women. Three women requested a higher dosage because of insufficient symptom relief, while one did not wish to continue taking pills. After the six month period 16 of the 17 women taking SH D A continued the treatment. Of the women taking SH D B, 7 continued SH D B, while 4 preferred a higher dosage and continued SH D A. One woman taking SH D A and 4 women taking SH D B were stopped because the drug was not available at that moment. *In the second study* all women finished treatment with SH D A and SH D B except 2, who stopped for non-drug-related causes.

Menopausal symptoms and side-effects

Flushes and night sweats were efficiently treated in most women, but 22%, 8% and 40% of women taking SH D A, SH D G and SH D B continued to have mild complaints after three months. In study I, mild dizziness was present in 20% of women taking SH D A and 29% of women taking SH D B: during treatment, this complaint occurred in 10% of women taking SH D B only. Insomnia, rated as severe in 33% and mild 22%, disappeared completely after 3 months of SH D A; rated as severe in 14% and mild in 43%, it continued as mild in 20% of women taking SH D B. Depression, scored as severe in 56% and mild in 11% before treatment disappeared completely after 4 cycles in SH D A; scored as severe in 29% and mild in 14%, it continued as mild in 10% of women taking SH D B. In study II, after 4 months of treatment with SH D A , dizziness rated initially as mild, moderate and severe in 33%, 27% and 13% of women dropped to 9% mild, insomnia dropped from 13%, 27%

and 20% respectively to 35% mild, depression dropped from 40%, 0% and 20% to 18% mild. After 4 months of treatment with SH D G dizziness dropped from 40% mild, 13% moderate and 13% severe to 8% mild and 15% moderate (NS), insomnia from 20%, 0% and 20% to 23% mild (NS) and depression from 33%, 27% and 7% to 0%. By two way analysis of variance (GLM) these effects were highly significant for hot flushes ($P < 0.0001$), night sweats ($P < 0.0001$), dizziness ($P < 0.0003$), insomnia ($P < 0.003$) and depression ($P < 0.0001$). Acne, hirsutism or seborrhea were not sufficiently frequently present to evaluate improvement.

No side-effects were noted, i. e. no headache, no varicosities, no edema, vomiting or nausea. Mild and severe breast tension was present in 9% and 18% of women taking SH D A, 5% and 12% of women taking SH D B and 15% and 7% of women taking SH D G respectively. Weight and blood pressure did not change during therapy (Tab. 2).

Hormone concentrations and general biochemistry were investigated during the first study only (Tab. 3, 4). After the intake of 2 mg estradiol valerate the plasma concentrations of 17β-estradiol and of estrone rose to 96 ± 35 and more than 400 pg/ml after 2 hours ($n = 6$) and to 67 ± 40 and 172 ± 104 pg/ml of 16 hours ($n = 15$). After the intake of 1 mg of estradiol valerate, the concentrations were 67 ± 31 and 243 ± 108 pg/ml ($n = 5$) and 36 ± 18 and 208 ± 102 pg/ml ($n = 6$) after 16 hours respectively. The concentrations of LH, FSH, prolactin, testosterone, androstenedione, cortisol, thyroid hormones and

Table 2. Weight and blood pressure (BP) before and during treatment (M ± SD)

Study I		Before	3 months	6 months
Weight	SH D A	57.2 ± 6.8	59.2 ± 6.7	58.6 ± 7.0
	SH D B	64.6 ± 10.7	65.9 ± 10.1	63.6 ± 11.6
Systolic BP	SH D A	131 ± 8	128 ± 13	129 ± 4
	SH D B	132 ± 13	133 ± 17	131 ± 18
Diastolic BP	SH D A	80 ± 7	78 ± 7	80 ± 5
	SH D B	79 ± 13	78 ± 13	76 ± 16
Study II		Before	3 months	6 months
Weight	SH D A	59.8 ± 6.6	62.6 ± 9.9	63.7 ± 7.8
	SH D B	62.2 ± 7.0	63.9 ± 8.1	63.3 ± 7.8
Systolic BP	SH D A	125 ± 5	119 ± 8	121 ± 6
	SH D B	122 ± 7	123 ± 10	121 ± 4
Diastolic BP	SH D A	77 ± 5	72 ± 8	79 ± 5
	SH D B	77 ± 5	78 ± 9	78 ± 4

Table 3: Hormone concentrations before and at the end of 3, 6 and 12 months of treatment with SH D A. Blood samples were taken fasting, 2–16 hours after tablet intake.

	Months of treatment			
	0	3	6	12
n	10	13	11	12
17β-estradiol (pg/ml)	50 ± 42	68 ± 28	72 ± 40	68 ± 52
Estrone (pg/ml)	70 ± 93	238 ± 146*	290 ± 130	196 ± 151
LH (mIU/ml)	24 ± 11	20 ± 9	24 ± 8	31 ± 20
FSH (mIU/ml)	41 ± 26	40 ± 23	36 ± 20	47 ± 18
PRL (μU/ml)	430 ± 750	160 ± 64	169 ± 128	133 ± 78
Testosterone (pg/ml)	306 ± 92	267 ± 111	258 ± 150	285 ± 106
Androstenedione (ng/ml)	1.07 ± 0.61	.92 ± .33	1.13 ± .63	.79 ± .37
Cortisol (mg%)	16 ± 7	16 ± 4	16 ± 6.	15 ± 5
T_4 (μg/ml)	8.5 ± 2.0	9.5 ± 2.2	9.6 ± 1.2	10.9 ± 3.0
T_3 (ng/ml)	128 ± 29	134 ± 59	130 ± 21	150 ± 18
TBG (mg/l)	20 ± 4	23 ± 4	21 ± 8	24 ± 2
SHBG (ng/100ml)	1.4 ± 1.4	2.9 ± 1.0*	2.8 ± 0.9**	3.4 ± 0.9*
Transcortin (mg/l)	48 ± 11	50 ± 14	46 ± 7	50.3 ± 12
1-25 OH Vitam. D (μU/ml)	39 ± 33	39 ± 19	49 ± 20	35 ± 13
Parathyr.horm. (pg/ml)	36 ± 9	47 ± 12	53 ± 9	43 ± 3

* $p < 0.01$, ** $P < 0.001$ versus pre-treatment M ± SD

of the binding proteins, transcortin and thyroid-binding-globulin remained virtually unchanged, at 3, 6 and 12 months for both therapies. A striking increase of sex-hormone-binding-globulin was, however, seen with treatment SHDA ($P < 0.001$).

Blood cell count, ionogram, liver function tests, renal function, iron and iron-binding capacity also remained unchanged during therapy (Tab. 5, 6).

Menstruation and endometrial histology (Tab. 7)

During treatment, the duration and amount of menstruation decreased ($P < 0.0001$) whereas the incidence of amenorrhea increased ($P = 0.0002$) progressively (ANOVA). Differences between treatment were observed only between SH D A and SH D B for amount of menstruation ($P = 0.01$) and incidence of amenorrhea ($P = 0.01$).

The endometrial biopsy taken before treatment confirmed the absence of ovarian function: insufficient material, atrophy or slight proliferation was

Table 4: Hormone concentrations before and at the end of 3 and 6 months of treatment with SH D B. Blood samples were taken fasting, 2–16 hours after tablet intake.

	Months of treatment		
	0	3	6
n	13	16	12
17β-estradiol (pg/ml)	31 ± 34	59 ± 62	52 ± 32
Estrone (pg/ml)	45 ± 42	181 ± 122	185 ± 54
LH (mIU/ml)	24 ± 13	25 ± 12	40 ± 29
FSH (mIU/ml)	47 ± 21	47 ± 21	48 ± 22
PRL (μU/ml)	182 ± 165	154 ± 66	112 ± 63
Testosterone (pg/ml)	255 ± 75	240 ± 89	220 ± 70
Androstenedione (ng/ml)	.85 ± .31	1.02 ± .35	.99 ± .29
Cortisol (mg%)	13 ± 6	15 ± 7	15 ± 3
T_4 (μg/ml)	8.5 ± 2.1	9.2 ± 2.7	8.1 ± 2.9
T_3 (ng/ml)	123 ± 24	127 ± 23	128 ± 24
TBG (mg/l)	21 ± 4	21 ± 3	22 ± 4
SHBG (ng/100ml)	1.7 ± 0.6	2.1 ± 0.7	2.0 ± 0.7
Transcortin (mg/l)	43 ± 7	42 ± 4	41 ± 4
1-25 OH Vitam. D (μU/ml)	27 ± 7	32.4 ± 14	42 ± 14
Parathyr.horm. (pg/ml)	41 ± 10	48 ± 12	54 ± 8

* $p < 0.01$ versus pre-treatment concentrations M ± SD

found in 6, 9 and 0 women using SH D B, in 4, 9 and 2 women taking SH D G, and in 5, 7 and 3, and in 5, 9 and 1 women using SH D A in study I and study II, respectively.

Endometrial histology was not significantly different when taken after 3, 6, 9, 12 and 15 months of therapy with SH D A (n = 10, 12, 3, 11 and 6 respectively) or SH D B (n = 10, 11, 2, 5 and 0 respectively). Therefore the different treatment periods were not analysed separately, and the duration of treatment was not taken into account in the analysis of variance. For the same reason, during the second study all biopsies were taken after 4 months of therapy. During the first study the endometrial biopsy was taken at random during the luteal phase, whereas during the second study, the endometrial biopsy was taken exactly on day 24 of a 28 day cycle.

During treatment the biopsy contained no and insufficient material in 14% and 57% during SH D B treatment (n = 35 biopsies), in 14% and 14% during SH D G (n = 14), and in 12% and 12%, and 8% and 0% during SH D A

Table 5: General biochemistry before and after 3, 6 and 12 months of treatment with SH D A (M ± SD).

	Months of treatment			
	0	3	6	12
n	9	13	11	11
Hemoglobin	13.5 ± 0.7	13 ± 0.6	13.4 ± 0.7	13.4 ± 0.5
Hematocrite	0.4 ± 0	0.4 ± 0	0.4 ± 0	0.4 ± 0.0
Leucocytes	6.6 ± 1.9	6.0 ± 1	6.0 ± 1.4	5.5 ± 1.1
Red blood cells (10^{12}/l)	4.4 ± 0.4	4.4 ± 0.3	4.5 ± 0.3	4.5 ± 0.2
Not segmented 1 (%)	1.2 ± 0.8	1.8 ± 1.4	1.5 ± 1.6	2.3 ± 1.9
Segmented 1 (%)	50 ± 10	53 ± 15	53 ± 11	58.1 ± 7.0
Eosinophils (%)	1.2 ± 0.8	1.7 ± 1.3	1.4 ± 1.2	1.0 ± 1.1
Basophils (%)	0	0.3 ± 0.5	0.4 ± 0.5	0.2 ± 0.4
Lymphocytes (%)	37 ± 9	35 ± 15	38 ± 9	34 ± 7.1
Monocytes (%)	11 ± 4	8 ± 4	6 ± 3	4.4 ± 1.5
Sodium (mEq/l)	142 ± 2	140 ± 1	139 ± 3	141 ± 1.9
Potassium (mEq/l)	4.3 ± 0.4	4.2 ± 0.9	4.2 ± 0.5	4.1 ± 0.3
Chloride (mEq/l)	104 ± 2	103 ± 3	104 ± 2	104.4 ± 2.1
HCO_3 (mEq/l)	27 ± 2.8	25.4 ± 1.5	24.2 ± 2.7	25.2 ± 2.1
Total protein (mcg/l)	17.3 ± 0.8	16.8 ± 1.2	17.4 ± 1.5	16.8 ± 0.7
BUN (mg/dl)	27 ± 4	27 ± 5	28 ± 7	27.4 ± 5.1
Urid acid (mg/dl)	3.8 ± 1.4	3.9 ± 0.9	4.4 ± 1.2	4.0 ± 0.9
Creatinine (mg/dl)	0.9 ± 0.2	0.9 ± 0.1	0.8 ± 0.2	0.9 ± 0.2
GOT (U/l)	13.4 ± 4	10 ± 3	12 ± 5	10.6 ± 3.0
GPT (U/l)	16 ± 10	10 ± 4	11 ± 6	10.0 ± 3.0
γGT (U/l)	31 ± 32.2	10 ± 7	9 ± 6	10.3 ± 7.1
Bilirubine direct (mg/dl)	0.5 ± 0.2	0.6 ± 0.3	0.5 ± 0.2	0.5 ± 0.1
Alcaline phosphatase (U/l)	111 ± 111	63 ± 23	64 ± 19	63.9 ± 21.6
Sedim. after 1 hour (mm)	4 ± 2	7 ± 6	7 ± 3	7.9 ± 6.0
2 hours (mm)	9 ± 5	13 ± 15	16 ± 7	19.8 ± 15.9
Iron (μG/dl)	125 ± 30	107 ± 31	110 ± 15	98 ± 27
Tot. Iron binding capacity (UG/dl)	365 ± 91	299 ± 47	335.7 ± 48	325.2 ± 52
Platelets (10^9/l)	305 ± 54	259 ± 76	256 ± 98	236 ± 15
Fibrinogen (g/l)	1.5 ± 0.2	1.7 ± 0.5	1.6 ± 0.3	1.9 ± 0.4

treatment (n = 40 and 13) in study I and II respectively. Biopsies taken during spotting or intermenstrual bleeding (3 during SH D A treatment and 1 during SH D B treatment) were not taken into account. Hyperplasia or adenomatous hyperplasia were not found in any of the biopsies. In those biopsies with sufficient material, the quality of the secretory phase was considered normal,

Table 6: General biochemistry before and after 3 and 6 months of treatment with SH D B (M ± SD).

	Months of treatment		
	0	3	6
n	13	16	11
Hemoglobin	13.4 ± 0.58	13.4 ± 0.7	13.5 ± 0.6
Hematocriet	0.4 ± 0	0.4 ± 0	0.4 ± 0
Leucocytes	6.0 ± 2.0	5.5 ± 1.7	5.2 ± 1.4
Red blood cells (10^{12}/l)	4.6 ± 0.3	4.6 ± 0.2	4.6 ± 0.3
Not segmented 1 (%)	1.6 ± 1.5	1.0 ± 1.2	3.1 ± 1.3
Segmented 1 (%)	56 ± 9	52 ± 9	52 ± 6
Eosinophils (%)	3.5 ± 2.4	1.7 ± 1.9	2.4 ± 2.4
Basophils (%)	0.4 ± 0.9	0.2 ± 0.4	0 ± 0.3
Lymphocytes (%)	32 ± 6	39 ± 9	36 ± 6
Monocytes (%)	7 ± 4	6 ± 5	7 ± 3
Sodium (mEq/l)	141 ± 2	140 ± 2	140 ± 2
Potassium (mEq/l)	4 ± 0.3	4 ± 0.3	3.9 ± 0.3
Chloride (mEq/l)	104 ± 2	104 ± 2	103 ± 2
HCO_3 (mEq/l)	26.2 ± 2	25.6 ± 1.7	25.9 ± 1.9
Total protein (mcg/l)	17 ± 1	17.1 ± 1.2	16.9 ± 0.8
BUN (mg/dl)	28 ± 5	28 ± 5	27 ± 6
Urid acid (mg/dl)	4.7 ± 1.3	4.1 ± 0.5	4.8 ± 1.2
Creatinine (mg/dl)	0.9 ± 0.1	0.8 ± 0.1	0.9 ± 0.1
GOT (U/l)	9 ± 3	9 ± 2	9 ± 1
GPT (U/l)	9 ± 2	10 ± 4	10 ± 4
γGT (U/l)	9 ± 4	11 ± 9	9 ± 5
Bilirubine direct (mg/dl)	0.6 ± 0.3	0.6 ± 0.3	0.5 ± 0.1
Alcaline phosphatase (U/l)	64 ± 15	62 ± 10	65 ± 14
Sedim. after 1 hour (mm)	11 ± 8	11 ± 8	12 ± 9
2 hours (mm)	24 ± 15	27 ± 18	28 ± 20
Iron (μG/dl)	110 ± 15	126 ± 38	110 ± 36
Tot. Iron binding capacity (UG/dl)	322.6 ± 26.6	318.9 ± 28	332 ± 34
Platelets (10^9/l)	332 ± 49	291 ± 70	310 ± 94
Fibrinogen (g/l)	1.7 ± 0.5	1.7 ± 0.4	1.8 ± 0.3

allowing dating in 80% of biopsies taken during SH D B in 46% (study I) and 62% (study II) taken during SH D A and in only 18% during SH D G. In the other biopsies dating was difficult because of irregular secretion. When dating was possible they coincided within 2 days with the day of the cycle in all women.

Table 7: Menstruation and cycle control: statistical significant differences are indicated for the duration of treatment (* P = 0.0001, ** P = 0.0002) and for the drug used (° P = 0.01, SH D A versus SH D B)

Cycle of treatment	1–2	3–4	5–6	2	4
	SH D A			SH D A	
Menstruation					
duration (days)*	3.9 ± 1.9	3.6 ± 1.8	3.1 ± 2.0	5.5 ± 1.1	4.5 ± 1.1
% scanty*°	33	35	52	15	36
% amenorrhea**°	12	21	25	7	9
% Spotting	8	27	7	0	18
	SH D B			SH D G	
Menstruation					
duration (days)*	3.4 ± 1.6	3.1 ± 2.2	1.4 ± 2.0*	5.1 ± 5.1	4.7 ± 1.0
% scanty*°	59	69	53	14	38
% amenorrhea**°	34	27	52	7	15
% Spotting	28	40	25	8	30

In order to evaluate more precisely the secretory transformation, each aspect was analyzed separately using visual analog scales. This was not performed in women treated with SH D B, because of the high incidence of insufficient material/endometrial atrophy.

In women treated with SH D A the secretory endometrial changes (Fig. 2–4) were comparable with those seen in the luteal phase of a normal menstrual

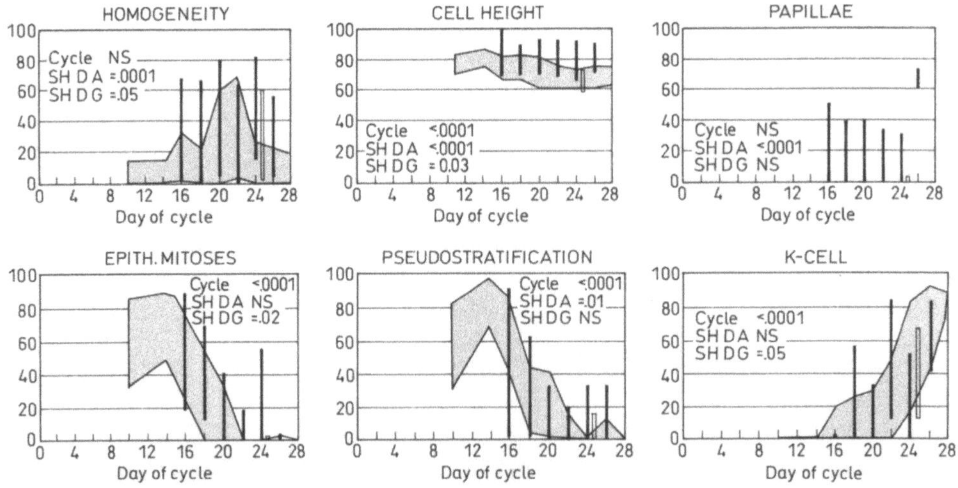

Fig. 2: Epithelial homogeneity, cell height, mitoses and pseudostratification, the formation of papillae, and the amount of K-cells in women treated with SH D A (■) or SH D G (□) in comparison with a normal menstrual cycle. Means ± 1 SD are depicted together with statistical significances.

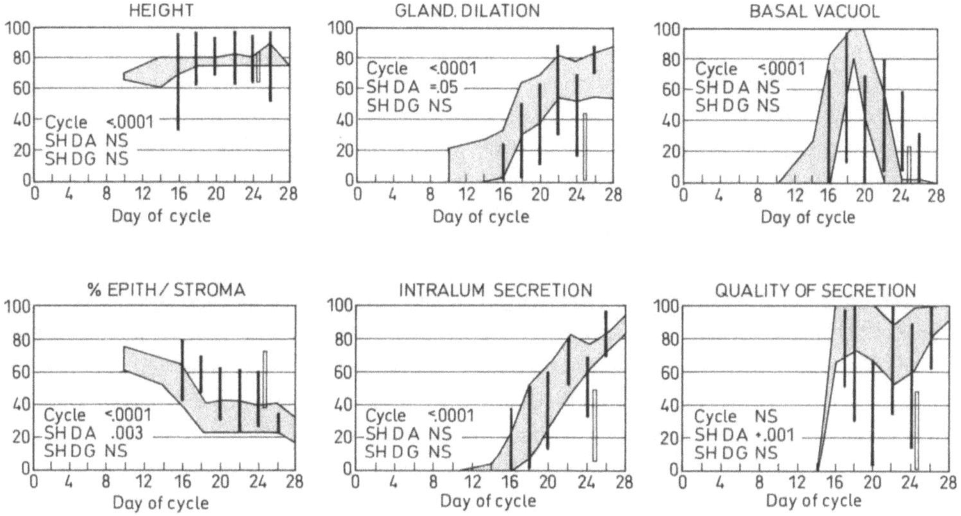

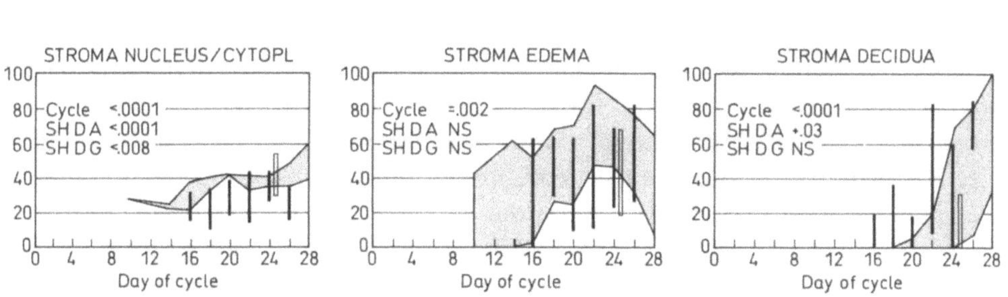

Fig. 4: Stromal mitoses, nuclear-cytoplasmic ratio, capillary dilatation, edema, spiral arteries and decidua in women treated with SH D A (■) or SH D G (□) in comparison with a normal menstrual cycle. Means ± 1 SD are depicted together with statistical significances.

cycle. Both glandular ($P < 0.001$) and stromal ($P = 0.04$) mitoses diminished gradually similar to a normal luteal phase. Basal vacuoles in the glandular epithelium developed normally on days 16 and 18 and disappeared in most biopsies between day 22 and 24 of the cycle. In women with irregular secretion (49%), basal vacuoles persisted in some glands up to day 24–26 of the cycle. Intraluminal secretion increased normally during the luteal phase, although glandular dilatation was slightly less ($P = 0.05$) and thus the epithelial/stromal ratio was slightly higher ($P = 0.003$) than in normal cycles.

The stromal cells were larger resulting in a decreased nuclear cytoplasmic ratio ($P < 0.0001$), whereas stromal decidua ($P = 0.03$) and fibrinoid material ($P = 0.001$) were more pronounced. Less ($P = 0.05$) spiral arteries were seen whereas stromal edema, capillary dilatation and the number of foam and K-cells were comparable with a normal menstrual cycle.

In women treated with SH D G only cross-sectional data were available on day 24 of the cycle. Endometrial secretion was comparable with a normal cycle and with those found in women treated with SH D A. The only significant differences with women treated with SH D A were: a more homogeneous epithelium ($P = 0.05$), less mitoses ($P = 0.02$) and a lower epithelial cell height ($P = 0.03$), slightly smaller stromal cells ($P = 0.006$) more K-cells ($P = 0.05$) and larger capillaries ($P = 0.05$).

Discussion

A drug designed for hormone replacement therapy should be effective in relieving menopausal symptoms, without unwanted side-effects. A sequential combination product should have a good cycle control, an amount and duration of menstruation which is acceptable for the patient, without endometrial hyperplasia and preferably with normal secretory changes. The product should furthermore prevent osteoporosis and cardiovascular accidents, and have a high mental tonic effect and a high patient acceptance. The sequential combination product SH D A was found to meet these criteria for effectiveness, patient acceptance, cycle control and endometrial effects. SH D A was highly effective in relieving menopausal complaints, not only for flushes and night sweats, but also for dizziness, insomnia and depression. No unwanted side-effects occurred. After 3 months most of the women had only a 'slight' menstruation for 3 days, whereas amenorrhea occurred in some 20%. In none of these patients was an hyperplastic endometrium found, while all evaluable biopsies taken at the end of the cycle showed good secretory changes. The patients' acceptance was high as evidenced by the high continuation rate. The only clinical side-effect was breast tenderness, whereas all biochemical parameters investigated remained normal.

The pill-free period of 7 days was often mentioned by the patient as too long: careful revision of the records failed to show, however, a consistent recurrence of menopausal symptoms during this period.

The high incidence of amenorrhea and scanty bleeding during SH D A can probably be related to the specific lipophilic characteristics of CPA, which accumulates in fat tissue, from where it is released over several days during the pill-free period. This is an advantage for most women who do not like abundant menstruations. The same mechanism is, however, probably responsible for the 10% breakthrough bleeding and/or spotting, generally during the follicular phase. In these women the endometriosis does not have sufficient time to proliferate, and this could explain the 10% 'atrophic' endometrial biopsies. In most women, however, the endometrium showed either a normal secretory transformation allowing dating, or an irregular secretion due to a strong progestogenic effect. In order to evaluate this progestogenic effect in greater detail, each parameter was scored on visual analog scales.

The evaluation of endometrial biopsies using visual analog scales yielded results which were astonishing comparable with those obtained by morphometry [8, 9]. The decline in glandular and stromal mitoses, the increase in glandular dilatation and intraluminal secretion, and the variability of these data were comparable with data obtained by morphometry. With all restrictions imposed by the qualitative and subjective evaluation in visual analog scales, this method seems to give satisfactory results, at least when performed by a well trained and experienced observer. Further studies will, however, be needed to evaluate the between-observer-variability, which was recently shown to account for 80% of the dating variability [4]. The visual analog scales have the advantage over morphometry of a much lower work load, making its use in large series feasible. We suggest that this method could be developed as the screening method of choice for evaluating endometrial effects, whereas morphometry could subsequently be used to confirm and quantitate unequivoqually the effects observed.

In the first study comparing 1 mg EV + 0.5 mg CPA (SH D B) with 2 mg EV + 1 mg CPA (SH D A), it was obvious that endometrial athropy and/or minimal proliferation together with amenorrhea and irregular spotting were a prominent feature of SH D B, whereas SH D A showed endometrial proliferation and secretion comparable with a normal menstrual cycle. Slight differences, such as a more irregular secretion, a more heterogeneous and higher glandular epithelium with more papillae, larger stromal cells, a more pronounced decidual reaction and more fibrinoid material, were interpreted as a strong progestagenic effect following a normal estrogen priming or as a normal progestagenic effect after a subnormal estrogenic priming. Since the normal height of the biopsy suggested a normal endometrial proliferation, a second study was performed in which 2 and 1 mg of CPA were compared. In order to achieve maximal statistical power, all biopsies were taken exactly on day 24 of the cycle, which is the last day of tablet intake. The differences observed were minimal and although some were statistically significant, the overall emerging picture was that the higher progestagen dose of 2 mg CPA did not improve endometrial secretory transformation, whereas some effects such as a decreased epithelial cell height and smaller stromal cells suggested an (unnecessary) strong progestagenic effect.

From these data it can be concluded that SH D A results in a normal endometrial proliferation and a normal secretory transformation in most women. In some women a marked progestagenic effect results in amenorrhea and irregular secretion. Since the bioavailability of oral steroid hormones is known to be variable, a high-normal progestagen dose can be considered to be an advantage in order to prevent endometrial hyperplasia and/or malignant transformation in all women.

SH D A, in comparison with SH D B and SH D G, is the product of choice. SH D B was clinically less effective for vasomotor symptoms, whereas cycle control was a problem in more than 20 percent. This could be related to the high incidence of endometrial atrophy. Our limited experience suggested, however, that SH D B could be useful for older age groups. SH D G had clinically similar effects as SH D A. The endometrial histology revealed, however, that 1 mg of CPA (SH D A) already had high progestagenic effects, which were only more pronounced with 2 mg CPA (SH D G).

In conclusion, SH D A is an excellent combination product for hormone replacement therapy since it is highly effective, with a high patient acceptance, since it has a good cycle control and limited bleeding during menstruation and because of physiologic progestagenic secretory effects upon the endometrium. The estrogen dose of SH D B is too low to be very effective for the treatment of vasomotor complaints, whereas the frequent occurrence of spotting is troublesome. SH D G is clinically undistinguishable from SH D A. A careful analysis of endometrial effects suggests, however, that the progestagenic effect of 1 mg CPA is already high enough which would make 2 mg CPA unnecessary unless anti-androgenic effects are intended.

Acknowledgments

Medgenix and Biomerieux are thanked for the generous supply of radioimmunoassay kits. Prof. E. Lesaffre is thanked for statistical advice, Dr B. Leysen is thanked for her help in study I. Mrs. M. Craessaerts co-ordinated these trials as a research nurse. Assays were taken care off by Mrs. C. Dewit. Mrs. D. Wolput prepared this manuscript and Mr. R. Ongkowidjojo made the designs, whereas Mr. Roels and Mr. Van Noppen are thanked for the photographs.

References

[1] Bouillon, R., H. van Baelen, P. De Moor: The measurement of the vitamin D-binding protein in human serum. J. Clin. Endocr. Metab. *45* (1977) 225.

[2] Dallenbach–Hellweg, G., H. Poulsen: Atlas of endometrial histopathology. Munksgaard, Copenhaegen 1985.

[3] Gambrell, Jr., R. D.: The menopause: benefits and risks of estrogen-progestogen replacement therapy. Fertil. Steril. *37* (1982) 457.

[4] Gibson, M., G. J. Badger, F. Byrn et al.: Error in histologic dating of secretory endometrium: variance component analysis. Fertil. Steril. *56* (1991) 242.

[5] Hammond, C. B., W. S. Maxson: Current status of estrogen therapy for the menopause. Fertil. Steril. *37* (1982) 5.

[6] Henderson, B. E., R. K. Ross, R. A. Lobo et al.: Re-evaluating the role of progestogen therapy after the menopause. Fertil. Steril. *49* (1988) 9 S.

[7] Heyns, W., P. De Moor: The binding of 17-hydroxy-5-α androstan-3-one to the steroid binding β-globulin in human plasma as studied by means of ammonium sulphate precipitation. Steroids *18* (1971) 709.

[8] Johannisson, E., B. Landgren, H. P. Rohr et al.: Endometrial morphology and peripheral hormone levels in women with regular menstrual cycles. Fertil. Steril. *48* (1987) 401.

[9] Johannisson, E., R. A. Parker, B. Landgran et al.: Morphometric analysis of the human endometrium in relation to peripheral hormone levels. Fertil. Steril. *38* (1982) 564.

[10] King, R. J. B., P. T. Townsend, N. C. Siddle et al.: Regulation of estrogen and progesterone receptor levels in epithelium and stroma from pre- and postmenopausal endometria. J. Steroid. Biochem. *16* (1982) 21.

[11] King, R. J. B., P. T. Townsend, M. I. Whitehead et al.: Biochemical analyses of separated epithelium and stroma from endometrium of premenopausal and postmenopausal women receiving estrogen and progestins. J. Steroid. Biochem. *14* (1981) 979.

[12] Koninckx, P. R., W. Heyns, G. Verhoeven et al.: Biochemical characterization of peritoneal fluid in women during the menstrual cycle. J. Clin. Endocr. Metab. *51* (1980) 1239.

[13] Lane, G., N. C. Siddle, T. A. Ryder et al.: Dose dependent effects of oral progesterone on the oestrogenised postmenopausal endometrium. Br. Med. J. *287* (1983) 1241.

[14] Lauritzen, C.: Clinical Use of Estrogens and Progestogens. Maturitas *12* (1990) 199.

[15] Noyes, R. N., A. T. Hertig, J. Rock: Dating the endometrial biopsy. Fertil. Steril. *1* (1950) 3.

[16] Paterson, M. E. L., T. Wade-Evans, D. W. Sturdee et al.: Endometrial disease after treatment with oestrogens and progestogens in the climacteric. Br. Med. J. *280* (1980) 822.

[17] SAS User's Guide: Statistics, Version 5, SAS Institute, Inc., SAS Campus Drive, P.O. Box 8000, Cary, North Carolina 27513–2414, 1985.

[18] Siddle, N. C., P. T. Townsend, O. Young et al.: Dose-dependent effects of synthetic progestins on the biochemistry of the estrogenized postmenopausal endometrium. Acta Obstet. Gynecol. Scand. *106* (1982) 17.

Bei Fragen zur Produktsicherheit wenden Sie sich bitte an:
If you have any questions regarding product safety,
please contact:

Walter de Gruyter GmbH
Genthiner Straße 13
10785 Berlin
productsafety@degruyterbrill.com